HEALTH CARE
TEAMWORK

HEALTH CARE TEAMWORK

Interdisciplinary Practice and Teaching

THERESA J. K. DRINKA AND
PHILLIP G. CLARK

Foreword by
DeWitt C. Baldwin, Jr., MD

AUBURN HOUSE
Westport, Connecticut • London

Library of Congress Cataloging-in-Publication Data

Drinka, Theresa J. K.
    Health care teamwork : interdisciplinary practice and teaching / Theresa J. K.
    Drinka and Phillip G. Clark ; foreword by DeWitt C. Baldwin.
       p. cm.
    Includes bibliographical references and index.
    ISBN 0–86569–297–1 (alk. paper)—ISBN 0–86569–298–X (paper : alk. paper)
    1. Health care teams. I. Clark, Phillip G. II. Title.
    R729.5.H4 D75   2000
    362.1′068—dc21   00–020903

British Library Cataloguing in Publication Data is available.

Library of Congress Catalog Card Number: 00–020903
ISBN: 0–86569–297–1
    0–86569–298–X (pbk.)

First published in 2000

Auburn House, 88 Post Road West, Westport, CT 06881
An imprint of Greenwood Publishing Group, Inc.
www.greenwood.com

Printed in the United States of America

The paper used in this book complies with the
Permanent Paper Standard issued by the National
Information Standards Organization (Z39.48–1984).

10 9 8 7 6 5 4 3 2 1

Contents

Illustrations

TABLES

FIGURES

Foreword

I am tempted to begin by saying that it has taken nearly a century for this book to be written. But such a provocative statement obviously demands an explanation.

As far as we know, the first formal proposals for assembling a team of health-related professionals to provide patient care in this country appeared in the early 1900s, when Richard Cabot, working in the Outpatient Department of the Massachusetts General Hospital, called for the "teamwork of the doctor, the educator, and the social worker."[1] This concept was echoed shortly thereafter by Michael Davis and Andrew Warner at the Boston Dispensary. It is of interest that these physicians all worked in outpatient departments, or what are now called ambulatory care clinics. Also, nurses were specifically not included in these teams. For one thing, at that time, nurses were not considered professionals; and, for another, their skills and contributions were still deemed to be subsumed under those of the physician. Finally, it is noteworthy that the impetus for the call for such teamwork arose not from patient care needs so much as from a professional concern— the threat of increasing specialization in medicine. All three of these physicians believed that the generalist physician was being gradually supplanted or displaced by the emerging specialists in medicine. Adding the social worker and the educator, then, was seen as assisting the specialist to maintain and preserve the broad social and educational perspectives of comprehensive patient care.

Despite this admirable, if hierarchically conceived, notion, the introduction of a concept such as interprofessional or interdisciplinary teamwork, especially for those whom we now refer to as ambulatory or primary care patients, was groundbreaking and significant.

Although the development of specialty-oriented, multidisciplinary, medical, surgical, and mental health teams became commonly accepted in the following decades, it took over half a century for the concept of interdisciplinary health care teams to become fully realized, as occurred during the community health center movement of the 1960s. In turn, this led to a major federal initiative to provide training for health professionals assigned to, or aspiring to become members of, the proposed primary care-oriented interdisciplinary health care teams. It took still another decade or two for such teams to be seen as essential in the care of a growing and poorly attended geriatric population.

So why did it take the rest of the century to produce this book? Largely, because it has taken that amount of time and experience to begin to separate the varying forms and functions of current and emerging interdisciplinary health care teams from their historical antecedents, and to be able to generalize about the specific and essential elements of teaming and teamwork in health care. It also required an important shift from the medical model of the first half century to the health care model of today.

Perhaps another way to elaborate on my provocative lead statement would be to look at this book from the standpoint of how persons involved at four key points in the development of interdisciplinary health care teams— in 1920, 1950, 1975, and 1999—would have viewed it.

In 1920, the theory and content of the book would have been virtually unintelligible to the authors of the initial proposals for teamwork. It would probably have been perceived and received with the same sense of incomprehension as were the interstellar rocket exploits of the cartoon strip character, Buck Rogers, nearly fifty years ago, or the wrist watch telephone of Dick Tracy—both of which have since become a reality. While the ideological values of better patient care would be shared, the pervading power and control of the medical profession and of the hospital clinic setting would have made the discussion of problems such as leadership and conflict appear irrelevant or absurd.

Even in 1950, it is doubtful if Martinsky and George saw their early community-based health care teams as much more than an immediate, innovative, practical way to deliver more effective medical care to address specific patient needs. Once again, the detailed discussion of values, leadership, decision making, relationships, power, and conflict elaborated by Theresa Drinka and Phillip Clark in these pages would not have been perceived as important or even relevant for a physician-led team. Even those of us who pioneered the early interdisciplinary educational endeavors of the time with their underlying ideological aims of egalitarianism viewed these efforts as logical and appropriate, but hardly generalizable to the entire spectrum of health professions education. It should also be noted that with the exception of George Szasz at the University of British Columbia, all these efforts occurred at the periphery of major institutional settings.

By 1975, the Community Health Center Movement had made the specific training of professionals for effective teamwork seem essential, but the theoretical models still came largely from the field of group dynamics and were heavily influenced by the ideologies of the time. The need to "prove" that the team concept was successful often precluded any systematic attempt to look more closely at the problems and processes of team care. The only seemingly egalitarian models came from the academically oriented team training programs funded by the government or the emerging use of teams in business. There were some real efforts to summarize and systematize the early experience and learnings of that time, some of which were quite sophisticated and deserve reexamination. Indeed, it is tragic that most of those communications have been essentially "lost" to the participants in the recent renewal of interest in interdisciplinary health care teams, partly because there were few, if any, venues for publishing that work and partly because the intent and focus of that phase of development was more on training and not on a broad spectrum of real-life, interdisciplinary health care team practice. Another way of putting it would be to say that the emphasis in 1975 was on the "team" as a unique, ideological construct, rather than the more realistic goal of efficient and cost-effective delivery of patient care. The constraints and demands of the environing health care systems were largely avoided by a focus on one specific component of care.

Today, as Drinka and Clark make clear, the emphasis has shifted to teams as desirable and appropriate means toward the end of better patient care—a focus on "means" rather than "ends." It fully accepts and deals with the arena of intrateam dynamics, as well as with that of the interface between the team and the dominant health care system. Equally important, it clearly distinguishes between interdisciplinary health care teams and the fashionable use of working teams in business and industry, while referencing the latter experience. As opposed to the highly structured, "set" teams of the 1970s—formed to meet predetermined and prescribed needs—modern interdisciplinary health care teams are more flexible, functional, and based on identifying realistic patient care and health professional needs as well as environing constraints.

Reading this book makes one aware of how far we have come. Indeed, one is reminded of a statement attributed to Anaïs Nin: "We don't see things as they are; we see things as we are." Perhaps, we are finally ready to see teams as they really are. For all of their frustrations and the "roller coaster" history of past and present interest and investment in interdisciplinary health care teams over the past fifty years, the current thrust, both on the campus and in practice, seems ready to take off and will be effectively guided by this timely and thorough contribution.

This is the book we have all been waiting for. It is broad, comprehensive, and practical, as well as a conceptual guide to teams and how to "team" with other health professionals in the service of a broader concept of patient care. Perhaps more importantly, the book focuses on the specific contributions to and problems of this process for the health professionals involved. Especially helpful and illuminating are the many tables listing detailed steps and concepts for consideration in team development and maintenance and the extensive use of clinically derived and oriented, real-time, and "real-team" illustrations. It should be required reading for anyone who is currently involved, or planning to become involved, with interdisciplinary health care teams, as well as for the health care administrators who must ultimately understand and support them.

DeWitt C. Baldwin, Jr., MD

NOTE

1. Baldwin, D. C. (1996). Some historical notes on interdisciplinary and interprofessional education in practice in health care in the USA. *Journal of Interprofessional Care*, 10, 173–187.

Acknowledgments

I would like to thank Professor Robert O. Ray for being a mentor and friend during the early development of this framework. I would also like to thank all of the team members across the country who have taught and inspired me. To my husband, Paul, I say thank you for your unending support, encouragement, and critical reviews. I would like to thank Cris for being my cheerleader. And finally, Jeni, I thank you for the insightful dialogue and for just being you.

—T.J.K.D.

Thanks to all my health professions colleagues over the years who have been real "team players" on the many educational and research projects on which we have collaborated. I have learned much from them about the perils, pitfalls, and payoffs of working together! And thanks also to the "home team"—Diana, Aaron, and Meredith—for your support and understanding. I am fortunate to have been blessed with such colleagues and family members!

—P.G.C.

Introduction

This book is about the practice and teaching implications of interdisciplinary health care teamwork. As such, it discusses a topic that has both an interesting and distinctive history and current relevance. As forces of change
sweep through the U.S. health care system, the subject of teamwork comes
to the forefront of discussion with renewed urgency.

   In the United States today, we are attempting to create systems of health
care delivery that provide the best care to the most people at the least cost.
However, as we face a new millennium, we find that in some ways health
care has not changed much in the last 100 years. In the year 2000, as in 1900,
a new era of technology is emerging; a tension exists in health care between
those who think that therapies should be research- and data-driven and
those who offer cures with herbal and other alternative remedies; and
nonphysician health care providers are struggling to redefine themselves,
resulting in independent channels of education and practice.

   Health care is plagued with mistakes that clinicians and administrators
try to cover up. Health care is as much a game of interpersonal communications as it is one of diagnosis and management. Harmful health care often
happens as a result of no communication or a breakdown in communication
between several providers who may or may not be from different disciplines
or between providers and patients. As health care systems hire less qualified

providers to cut costs, they may not put sufficient resources into training the lesser skilled to do the job. Even if the technical skills are in place, the interactional and team skills are not. There is no time, money, or expectation supporting the more highly skilled providers to interact with and teach the lesser skilled providers, especially across disciplines. There is only limited time to review the results of care. The development and maintenance of interdisciplinary health care teams (IHCTs) may be the best solution to fragmented, mistake-ridden health care. However, this cannot be the 1980s version of "everyone (including the janitor) sitting around a table" team. This is not the administrator's "business school vision" of team, nor is it the health providers "stick together with your own kind" vision of team.

If interdisciplinary teams are to thrive, they must become lean, efficient, and sophisticated entities for health care delivery. The individual member, the team, and the organization all share responsibility for accomplishing this. It is not sufficient to promote initial team development training and then leave the team on its own to function or to try to deliver care as an interrelated system. It is equally important to develop and learn the team system, recognizing that such a sophisticated system needs to be maintained, and that team members must be allowed time and must take time to manage their team.

Although this book includes some organizational and patient care perspectives, it focuses on the team members and the inner workings of the team. As authors, we have tried to remain unbiased. However, that is impossible. This book is colored by our experiences as clinicians, educators, researchers, and administrators. Our perspectives relate to what to call the team, what to call the recipients of care, patients as team members, the use of models, the interdisciplinary team approach to health care, and how this book might be used.

WHAT TO CALL THE TEAM

We struggled with what to call the kind of teams about which we are writing and settled on the term *interdisciplinary*. We considered using the term *interprofessional*, but realized early on that this term is limiting in the sense that the team might consist of more than just professionals (e.g., nursing assistants, technicians, or other community support systems). There is debate about which disciplines should be considered professionals and we did not want to enter that debate. We could have used the term *collaborative*, but it is not always essential for team members to collaborate because in many situations team members must practice autonomously. Thus, we decided on the term *interdisciplinary* more for its inclusiveness than anything else. Interdisciplinary is a term that has been around for a long time. If it does not describe what people want it to describe, we believe that is because many authors have not defined their terms and over time this word has come to take on meanings that were not intended. We have defined our use of it and use it throughout the book.

WHAT TO CALL THE RECIPIENT OF CARE

We were not sure what to call the people who come to health care providers for service. With the advent of the consumer movement and managed care organizations, terminology has developed intending to establish a person's involvement in his or her care (e.g., customer, consumer, client, participant, and partner to name a few). We decided to use the term *patient* because, historically, it designates the primary focus for a health care intervention. We firmly believe that patients must be involved in determining their course of health care.

PATIENTS AS TEAM PARTICIPANTS

Although we believe that patients should be actively involved in their care, we also believe that patients should be active according to their abilities. The responsibility of the patient, his or her advocate, or both to express the patient's needs and desires is not only difficult, but it is demanding when the patient does not feel good or is mentally unstable. Determining a patient's true mental and physical capability for participation can be very difficult and is one of the responsibilities of the highly skilled health care provider or health care team. We believe that the patient's needs are central to the team's focus and a patient or designee must be an active participant in the team's work. However, it is disingenuous to consider the patient a member of an interdisciplinary health care team that needs to work on its tasks and processes for health care delivery.

THE USE OF MODELS

This book is filled with models. It is our belief that you cannot travel to a place that is obscure and unknown without a road map. We see interdisciplinary health care teams as obscure and unknown and the models provided as road maps. Roads change and maps are reissued from time to time. It is our intention that these models provide fuel for dialogue and debate and that they will evolve as our knowledge of IHCTs continues to evolve.

Understanding the models that are presented in this book will help you to understand key principles behind interdisciplinary teamwork. The structures and forms of health care teams will continue to evolve, and they will require innovative methods and processes. Rather than presenting lists of methods and processes, we felt that it was more important to understand the principles and elements of successful interdisciplinary teamwork so that you can adapt them to new team structures and create methods that will work in those structures.

We also intend for you to challenge the models as you progress in your learning about teamwork. It is our hope that this book will prompt you to initiate small or large research projects to examine whether or not an element of teamwork really works. The ideas and models presented in this book reflect our collective knowledge of interdisciplinary teams. That knowledge continues to grow. As you grow in your knowledge of teamwork, we encourage you to help others to understand the principles as well.

THE INTERDISCIPLINARY TEAM APPROACH TO HEALTH CARE

There are those who equate teams with groups and those who recognize teams but do not distinguish between different types of teams. Group development or organizational development theory is applied, by some, to all small groups. This has contributed to the scarcity of funding for research on the development and function of different kinds of teams and groups. If we reduce all teams to groups and all groups are thought to be the same, then there is no point in comparing different kinds of groups or teams. This book is based on the assumption that groups may be a part of but are not the same as teams; that health care teams are different from other kinds of business teams; and that there are different kinds of health care teams. The health care teams that we write about in this book are IHCTs.

Neither every type of patient nor every situation calls for a team approach. Well-developed and efficient teams are those that can quickly evaluate a complex situation and decide how to state the problem so the members of the team can use their skills to focus on an integrated approach. Members participate only when and how they are needed. This type of team requires more initial effort and pays off in the long term. It pays off if the system is stable enough to allow teams to develop around a core element of trust. It is only through mutual trust that errors will be noted as problems to be solved and processes to be improved.

To work, a new vision of *team* must come from the heart of health care, not just from the educators, clinicians, or administrators. In order to work, interdisciplinary teamwork must become part of the fabric of health care. As the world begins a new millennium, managed care is struggling for dominance in the U.S. health care arena. The current bottom-line focus of health care is the controlling force that is keeping teams from treating the person holistically. The problem is that the bottom line that administrators and investors view is not the real bottom line. The monetary bottom line does not account for many of the problems that make the current health care system distasteful to many and untenable to those who have been hurt or shortchanged by it. We expect doctors to be "know-all gods" in an environment where knowledge is exploding and the time allowed with patients is imploding. Instead, we must tap the potential of all health care professionals to solve complex problems of patients and the common and uncommon complex problems of health care. We ask the readers to reflect on these issues, just as many of the current health professions have hunkered down to protect their individual domains.

We call health care a business. Business literature is full of messages about the "learning organization." In the learning organization, employees at all levels not only learn continuously, but they actively seek new ways to apply their knowledge to help the company, and themselves, reach and exceed their goals. Unfortunately, health care does not have a common goal. The funders, administrators, providers, patients, and educators appear to have separate goals. So, where is the learning in the health care organization? We keep hearing about health care organizations cutting back on patient care meetings for teams, moving learning conferences to early morning prebusiness hours, and reducing opportunities for health care providers to collaborate. So what is the real message? Are these mixed messages the result of not understanding IHCTs; are health care administrators afraid of learning organizations; or do health care organizations really not want a team approach to health care? We begin this book by placing these questions on the table as stimuli for open dialogue between health care providers, educators, administrators, funders, and patients.

I

Are Health Care Teams
What We Think They Are?

An interdisciplinary health care team (IHCT)—consisting of a nurse, physician, nurse practitioner, and social worker—is operating a primary care clinic in the inner core of a large city. Like most primary care clinics, its patients are a mix of relatively healthy individuals and the walking wounded. Many of the patients, like Mrs. Adams, have physical problems that periodically are accompanied by grief, anxiety, or depression. Patients' problems are often coupled with a history of low unstable income and pressing family responsibilities. Some of the families have been struggling with serious mental health or substance abuse issues. Mrs. Adams is now the caregiver for her husband who, at the age of 52, has just been diagnosed with Alzheimer's disease. She has been the primary caregiver for her 3-year-old grandson while her daughter looks for work.

Mrs. Adams has adult onset diabetes and rheumatoid arthritis. She has recently been treated for an episode of major depression. Through close collaboration, the clinic team has been managing Mrs. Adams' problems by making and monitoring changes in her medications, instructing her on joint protection as she takes on new tasks, and helping her find a day-care center for her husband. The members of the team have fielded numerous calls from Mrs. Adams in the past 2 weeks. As the events with her husband unfolded, Mrs. Adams had a serious flare-up of her arthritis and communication among the team members increased to try to address the problems before they resulted in her incapacitation. The team added Mrs. Adams' name to the list of patients to discuss at their weekly care-planning meeting.

Last month, a large managed care organization purchased the hospital that funds the clinic serving Mrs. Adams. Yesterday, the new administrator requested that the team physician attend a meeting to discuss the clinic operation. Subsequently, at the weekly care-planning meeting, the physician announced that the administrator had stated that the clinic was in financial trouble and that all of the clinics in the facility had to increase their efficiency. However, the administrator was particularly concerned with this clinic's lack of efficiency because it was using a team model that was "inherently inefficient." The administrator said it was imperative to find ways to cut back and suggested that the team clinic stop its weekly meetings, which would allow each team member to schedule four more patients per day. The team members were stunned and were not sure how they would defend their team clinic operation. The rest of the care-planning meeting was very difficult and each member of the team went home that evening feeling disheartened.

The next day, the clinic social worker and the nurse practitioner wanted to meet with the administrator to defend the need for a team in the clinic. The clinic nurse said that she was afraid to speak up for fear of losing her job. The team physician said that the managed care organization was measuring clinic productivity by the number of patient visits and that the clinic's productivity would be reflected in the team members' pay. He felt that they should just accept the decision because they did not have a chance of changing the philosophy of the new administration. Some of the team members were not sure if they wanted to continue working for the clinic and others decided to keep quiet for fear of losing their jobs.

This case is an example of the interrelated clinical and social issues that create complexity in health care. The vignette also represents changes and dilemmas that are occurring in health care and the confusion among health care providers. Health care teams are forced to defend their positions as they are learning to cope with new systems of care and the changing philosophies of management. Yet, health care providers retain an innate sense that they cannot always provide care alone or without formal mechanisms for collaboration.

Each of us has encountered situations in which we have tried to solve a complex problem with only part of the knowledge necessary to do so. Sometimes we are unaware of our deficits and continue in our solo attempts. Later, we realize that the solution will require knowledge that we do not have and do not have time to acquire. In clinical health care settings, these dilemmas are common. In fact, we are bombarded by these situations. To address some of these dilemmas, wise health care providers elicit the help of others with appropriate knowledge, perhaps a professional from another discipline, an administrator, or a member of the support staff. However, when similar or complex problems arise frequently, those we ask for help might become irritated or resentful that we are asking so much of their time when they have their own jobs to do. This signals that the consultation process may be inefficient for these problems and that a more formal team effort with established expectations, goals, procedures, and responsibilities might produce better results.

Unfortunately, most clinical health care providers were trained in their own autonomous health professions and were not formally taught a foundation for team practice. Health providers begin working on teams because they realize that they cannot provide care alone for some patients. Clinicians' intelligence and experience tells them that they need the help of professionals with different skills to provide care for patients who have complex problems. As clinicians begin to interact more closely with other care providers they realize that providers from different disciplines have philosophies that differ from theirs. Few team members are prepared to address the language differences, the inevitable conflict issues, the different problem-solving styles, and the systems issues that teamwork brings. Without a context for decision making, it is difficult for health care providers who are from different fields with different ways of thinking to dialogue effectively for the benefit of the patient. This is why complex health care situations require formal structures and processes that efficiently and effectively use the talents of individuals from different disciplines.

IHCTs are not just assemblages of individuals from different professions. They are complex and paradoxical entities that often seem to defy understanding. Team situations that appear easy and straightforward are not. Individuals who preach teamwork are not always willing to support it. Teams that seem to be developed and well functioning may be full of camouflaged chaos. And, teams that seem chaotic and dysfunctional may actually be creating a unique solution to a vexing problem. Despite these paradoxes, and perhaps because of them, well-functioning IHCTs continue to make sense for the emerging health care systems. We believe that one can effectively use only what one truly understands. It follows that if health care providers do not fully understand teams, they will not be able to create efficient ones, nor defend their teams to administrators. In this chapter, we begin to explore a common understanding of IHCTs by reviewing some definitions and a brief history of health care teams.

DEFINITIONS OF TEAMS AND GROUPS: A MUDDLE OF TERMINOLOGY

Let's get a team to work on this! Let's call ourselves a team! We make the best team! The power of teamwork! Because working together is a part of the human experience, the simple word *team* has become a catchword for a group of people who are designated as working together in some capacity (e.g., teaching team, health care team, sports team, project team, self-directed team). The word *team* is commonly applied to many different types of teams and methods of work. In reality, the undescribed entity *team* could have an almost infinite number of variables. A team could have 2 members or 20, be temporary or permanent, provide ongoing care or merely perform assessments, be recently assembled or long term, contain all experts or all generalists, have all members of the same discipline or of many disciplines; or have members who are solely assigned to one team or many teams. Within this broad context, there is an array of potential meanings that render the term *team* unusable if it is not accompanied by a specific definition.

Health care teams have been described as multidisciplinary, interdisciplinary, cross-disciplinary, polydisciplinary, pandisciplinary, transdisciplinary, and virtual. Unfortunately, these terms are often used interchangeably to refer to *team*. Perhaps it is because the word *team* encompasses so many variables that it is often reduced to the least common denominator. When an entity is too complex to understand, simplifying its use affords people a way to cope with it. One of the drawbacks to simplifying the expression *team* is that health care providers and health administrators often assume understanding when they may be discussing different entities. It is common for physicians to equate health care teams with a group of physicians from different specialties. Health professionals who have very little contact with each other may refer to themselves as a team or be referred to as a team.

In an effort to determine the extent of the problem of misusing the term *health care team* in the field of geriatrics, Drinka and Ray[1] conducted a cross-sectional review of the geriatrics literature for any articles that related to health care teams. The review covered the years 1982, 1986, and 1990. This review revealed that although most articles were descriptive with the intent of teaching general geriatrics, the teams were not well described. Physician-directed patient outcome studies of acute care consult teams appeared to be increasing without adequate descriptors of the independent variable that was the team. Also, consult teams may have been the least likely type of team to benefit elderly patients, and yet, in the early 1990s, these acute care teams (without description) represented the majority being reported in the geriatrics literature. These articles were in journals directed to physicians, the discipline with the most influence in health care systems. Unfortunately, much of the literature on IHCTs that was published during the subsequent decade does not appear to be any better at defining terms, clarifying meaning, or using consistent terminology.

Overgeneralization of the team concept may cause team members to assume that merely assembling a group of nice people will render team building unnecessary. Health professionals justify that generalization by correctly asserting that they are very busy with the important work of caring for people. Their incorrect corollary to that assertion is assuming that they do not have time for team building, which they view as less important than delivering health care. Health care administrators support health care professionals in both assertions by expecting them to work ever harder to increase efficiency in health care services. Because administrators and professionals do not necessarily see immediate results from team building, they tend not to trust it and often do not ensure that it takes place.

Identifying a group of people and calling them a team does not mean that they function well or at all as a team. Nice people may behave very differently in a team than they do either individually or in a small group. And, because most health professionals have been trained to function autonomously they may have difficulty with teams. Although it is easy to imagine a virtual team that has most contacts by telephone, e-mail, or satellite hook-ups, it is difficult to imagine a functioning team that has neither developed its processes and structures for communication nor established methods for evaluation. Establishing processes, structures, and methods for evaluation takes work and that is the "stuff" of teams that is rarely spoken of and is often left to chance. Subsequently, when teams experience trouble they either obtain help; limp along until they dissolve; or become so inefficient that the organization eventually "reorganizes" and puts them out of their misery.

A DEFINITION OF INTERDISCIPLINARY HEALTH CARE TEAM

Because the function and structure of an IHCT can have an impact on the type of care that is delivered, studies involving health care teams should contain adequate descriptors of the team variable. This is important because different types of teams have different costs and benefits and produce different outcomes. Another reason why it is important to use the terminology of teams correctly—or at least to define the terminology that is being used—is because a common understanding helps people communicate more efficiently with greater accuracy. In a field that has been so misunderstood, use of commonly understood terminology is critical to gaining credibility. Unfortunately, the problem with ill-defined IHCTs has been a force for so long, that it is unlikely that a common definition will be achieved in the near future. However, this does not excuse us from stating our definitions.

For the purposes of this book, an IHCT is defined as follows:

An IHCT integrates a group of individuals with diverse training and backgrounds who work together as an identified unit or system. Team members consistently collaborate to solve patient problems that are too complex to be solved by one discipline or many disciplines in sequence. In order to provide care as efficiently as possible, an IHCT creates formal and informal structures that encourage collaborative problem solving. Team members determine the team's mission and common goals; work interdependently to define and treat patient problems; and learn to accept and capitalize on disciplinary differences, differential power, and overlapping roles. To accomplish these they share leadership that is appropriate to the presenting problem and promote the use of differences for confrontation and collaboration. They also use differences of opinion and problems to evaluate the team's work and its development.

The concept of a functional unit is particularly important because it allows for a continuously evolving core operation for evaluation, feedback, and improvement.

At the most basic level, teamwork relies on the ability of team members to communicate with one another. If practitioners are not sure who is on the team and they are a member of the team it is difficult to know what, how, when, or with whom to communicate. Also, if the team has not agreed on what needs to be communicated, there will be disparate views about what information to pass on to other members—which members and in what format. The more that IHCTs leave cross-discipline communication to chance or restrict it to formal occasions, the more likely it is that communication will not happen when the complexity and seriousness of a situation call for it.

EMERGENCE OF INTERDISCIPLINARY TEAMWORK AS A SCIENCE

Appreciating the value of IHCTs has been an off-and-on phenomenon for much of the 20th century. Although the process appears to be slow at times, with each wave of interest the principles and theory of IHCTs continue to evolve. In the early part of the 20th century, many physicians worked from their homes and a physician's wife might have worked with her husband as a team, functioning as office nurse and secretary. With increased regulation of medical schools and the publication of the *Flexner Report* in 1910, medicine as the embodiment of health care became a scientific pursuit. Subsequently, the human touch may have lost value as a necessary part of a person's health care.[2] To fill this void and to address other areas of health care, new health professions emerged. Also, despite medicine's primary focus on science and technology during most of the 20th century, many physicians continued to deliver primary care and were familiar with their patients' physical and emotional health. Because they were trained to practice autonomously, physicians and other disciplines worked side by side in a sequential and sometimes contradictory fashion.

An organized form of IHCT originated in the 1940s when Montefiore Hospital in New York City started a hospital-based home care program that was staffed by a team of health professionals.[3] Health care teams have continued to emerge in every decade since that time and interdisciplinary thinking has evolved with them. In the 1950s, the interdisciplinary idea progressed in the area of Family Health at Montefiore[4] and the University of Washington.[5] Both settings used IHCTs to deliver comprehensive patient care and the University of Washington used an interdisciplinary team of faculty to teach team care to students from different disciplines.

The development of IHCTs was advanced in the 1960s during the era of the "Great Society" with Neighborhood Health Centers, funded by the federal Office of Economic Opportunity. Members of eight teams, which were created by the Martin Luther King, Jr. Neighborhood Health Care Center in New York, included physicians and nurses plus community health workers.[6] Until this time, little was written about the inner workings of IHCTs. The Neighborhood Health Center teams originally had social workers as part of their core. The health care professionals thought of the social workers as irritants and eventually replaced them with untrained health workers. The result was a lack of team growth and a loss of the knowledge base that social work might have brought to the health centers. Although the Neighborhood Health Center teams were trained using methods developed for teams in business organizations, little was done to understand the clash of cultures among the social workers, nurses, and physicians.

In the mid-1970s and again in the late 1980s the Veterans Administration and the Bureau of Health Professions of the U.S. Public Health Service supported universities in the development of IHCT training. From the mid-1970s through the 1990s the U.S. Department of Veterans Affairs supported the development of Interdisciplinary Team Training Programs (ITTP). Although the programs differed in structure and content, they trained hundreds of health professions' students in how to work with other disciplines in delivering care to populations with complex problems (e.g., geriatrics, mental health, rehabilitation, and primary care). Also in the late 1980s, the Division of Associated, Dental, and Public Health Professions began funding initiatives for interdisciplinary health team training in rural areas.[7]

In the late 1990s, the John A. Hartford Foundation funded 3-year grants for Geriatric Interdisciplinary Team Training (GITT) Programs in managed care settings. The Hartford Foundation's Programs also experienced many successes as they trained hundreds of health professions' students in different models of team-delivered care. Additionally, they introduced managed care systems to interdisciplinary practice.

Unfortunately, in each of these endeavors, some of those who were expected to teach interdisciplinary care had never been formally trained or had received only basic training in the theory of IHCT development and maintenance. This is the catch-22 of teaching IHCT theory and practice. In general, educational and health care organizations devote little time and resources to developing the science of IHCTs. Because of this neglect, health care providers often function in various groups that purport to be interdisciplinary but in fact are only groups masquerading as IHCTs. Myths that teams hold of being "a good team" help to perpetuate this culture and may prevent the growth of interdisciplinary practice. The knowledge that many practicing health care providers have of IHCTs may never grow beyond their formal training, if in fact they ever received any training in IHCT theory and function. Educational institutions and health care organizations must help structure and support continuing development and maintenance activities for IHCTs in order to break through the catch-22 of having health care providers, who are poorly trained in IHCT function, train new health care providers.

Evidence of the growing support for greater interdisciplinary collaboration and teamwork has been articulated recently by several national organizations and commissions, as follows here:

- The Joint Commission on the Accreditation of Health Care Organizations (JCAHO) now requires evidence of interdisciplinary collaboration in hospitals, nursing homes, and clinics as part of its accreditation review process.

- The report of the President's Advisory Commission on Consumer Protection and Quality in the Health Care Industry has explicitly recommended that "the training of physicians, nurses, and other health care workers should provide those individuals with greater experience in working in interdisciplinary teams."

- The American Association of Colleges of Nursing has released an official position statement in support of interdisciplinary education and practice for nurses.

- The Bureau of Health Professions of the U.S. Public Health Service has officially recommended the development of interdisciplinary training experiences and curricula in geriatrics.

- The American Geriatrics Society has recommended the inclusion of interdisciplinary training in the curriculum for medical residents.

- The National Committee for Quality Assurance Standards for Accrediting Health Plans and behavioral health managed care organizations require coordination of care between primary care physicians and behavioral health practitioners.

SUMMARY

This chapter has provided a working definition of an IHCT, which can serve as the basis for discussion and evaluation of other team definitions. It sometimes seems as though there are as many definitions for teams as there are teams. In discussing IHCTs with others, having the "one true definition" is not as important as providing a definition. Hopefully, this chapter prompts you to ask questions when team definitions are assumed and not made explicit. Sharing definitions is the first step in promoting true dialogue about IHCTs. Through this dialogue, health care providers will establish a foundation from which to advance the science of IHCTs and create functional models for training, practice, and research. The chapter has also provided a brief outline of some of the history of IHCTs, which should help you to question why the understanding of health care teams has not progressed further since the 1940s. This brief review also provides hope for the future of IHCTs. Despite the sparseness of good working team models and the paucity of funding for research, IHCTs have survived. Despite the heightened interest in making health care a profitable enterprise, the lure of interdisciplinary health care remains, especially in the expanding areas of outpatient and community health care. Increasingly, health care professionals know that they cannot provide good care for all patients through autonomous practice. Some also realize that they cannot provide efficient care for complex problems through consultation models. There is evidence that new initiatives for funding projects in interdisciplinary care and education are based on learning that occurred in previous interdisciplinary efforts. Hopefully, this learning will propel us forward and keep us from repeating the mistakes of our collective past.

NOTES

1. Drinka, T.J.K., & Ray, R. O. (1992). Health care team ≠ Health care team. In J. R. Snyder (Ed.), *Proceedings of the fourteenth annual conference on inter-*

disciplinary health care teams (pp. 1–12). Indianapolis: School of Allied Health Sciences, Indiana University Medical Center.

2. Starr, P. (1982). *The social transformation of American medicine.* New York: Basic Books.

3. Cherkasky, M. (1949). The Montefiore hospital home care program. *American Journal of Public Health, 39,* 163–166.

4. Silver, G. (1958). Beyond general practice: The health team. *Yale Journal of Biology and Medicine, 31,* 29–38.

5. Deisher, R. W. (1953). Use of the child health conference in the training of medical students. *Pediatrics, 11,* 538–543.

6. Wise, H., Beckhard, R., Rubin, I., & Kyte, A. (1974). *Making health teams work.* Cambridge, MA: Ballinger.

7. Baldwin, D. C. (1996). Some historical notes on interdisciplinary and interprofessional education and practice in health care in the USA. *Journal of Interprofessional Care, 10,* 173–187.

2

Developing and Maintaining Interdisciplinary Health Care Teams

Defining IHCTs is only a beginning. The primary care clinic team introduced in chapter 1 was facing some problems that were complex, interrelated, and indefinite. These types of problems, like addressing the needs of an ill caregiver when those needs conflict with the needs of an ill spouse, require complex solutions. Some complex problems are common and if identified as such, members can construct policies and procedures to increase their efficiency in addressing these problems. However, many complex problems are uncommon and providing complex solutions can be costly in terms of staff time and effort. Thus it is important to establish an IHCT that can improvise and effectively use the most appropriate resources that it has to offer. This chapter provides a model for understanding IHCTs as the complex, dynamic, and useful entities that they are. The first three sections outline a conceptual framework that captures the necessary components and patterns of development within an IHCT. The final section addresses the efficiency of interdisciplinary practice. This model was developed over a period of 20 years and has been tested in an ongoing IHCT.[1] It explains how IHCTs must develop and work in order to solve the types of problems for which they are created. This chapter shows how IHCTs that are well developed can be efficient vehicles for delivering health care in a wide range of situations. Finally, this chapter explains that IHCTs differ from other types of teams and must be recognized as the distinct entities that they are.

FOUR ESSENTIAL TEAM COMPONENTS AND
THEIR VARIABLES

An understanding of the dynamics of IHCTs does not come naturally for most people. One review of team research noted that team training in the process area has little effect on improving outcomes but that focusing on goals does.[2] In our experience, an IHCT can focus on its goals but unless it is also aware of its dynamics, the team's long-term outcomes will be adversely affected.

An IHCT is made up of essential components that should work together to achieve the team's goals in an effective and efficient manner. Understanding how a team's components and their variables are working together is complex and this makes it difficult to diagnose team function and dysfunction.

The organization and the team share responsibility for assuring that the individual and professional practice components are in place and appropriate for the team's work. The team has internal cultural components that it cultivates through goal setting, problem solving, and conflict management. These require the team to establish appropriate structure and process. The broader organization works with the team to provide the resources to accomplish the team's mission and to keep it aligned with the mission of the organization. Finally, the team maintains itself in a growth pattern through learning, leadership, and teaching. These four components are necessary for an IHCT to thrive. However, some components may be neglected, and that neglect can lead to problems in the team's ability to develop effectively. The variables encompassed by these components are ever changing and interacting. The components of an IHCT form the base of the team development model. Understanding these components (Table 2.1) will help team members determine where the problems lie when a team is malfunctioning.

Practice Components: Personal and Professional

Although personal characteristics are downplayed, they perform a major role during the initial formation of an IHCT or following significant changes in focus or membership. The ongoing impact of personal factors on a team's members is unique to each team and although personal characteristics such as charisma may not be a significant source of power in an existing IHCT, they do affect a team's function.[3] The greatest impact of personal characteristics might be when new members enter an IHCT that is already developed. In this situation, the personal factors of age, gender, cultural background, styles of relating, and charisma of members are the magnet that attracts a new member to an existing member. This attraction may be an important factor in the type of orientation a new member receives. The results will de-

Table 2.1

The Interdisciplinary Health Care Team: Components and Variables

I. Issues That Directly Influence Practice

Personal
•age/gender/culture
•communication skills
•energy
•styles of relating
•willingness to risk/flexibility
•leadership styles
•openness to new knowledge
•personal knowledge/maturity
•self-respect
•awareness of personal conflict styles

Professional
•expertise in specialty
•dedication to an ideal
•respect for professional differences
•broad knowledge of health care
•willingness to share client
•professional maturity
•knowledge of roles of others
•knowledge of systems
•knowledge of ways different professionals
   problem solve

II. Intra Team Issues

Team Structure
•formal leadership
•norms
•composition
•formal professional roles
•team culture
•professional status
•physical placement
•structure for interaction
•structure for innovation

Team Process
•negotiating informal leadership
•goal setting
•appreciating values
•negotiating team roles
•building trust
•communicating
•problem setting
•problem solving/influencing
•managing conflict

III. Organizational Issues

Internal Organization
•philosophy re: teams
•resource allocation
•rigid vs. flexible rules
•simple/complex structure

External Organization
•national policy
•funding sources
•philosophy
•interdisciplinary values

IV. Actions Necessary For Team Maintenance Over Time

Team
•members use power for decision making
•all commit to freedom of dissent
•members willing to resolve conflict
•team evaluates and manages itself
•ongoing members teach leadership to new
   members

Organization
•communicates organization's mission to the team
•uses team feedback to revise mission
•allows the team to manage itself
•gives constructive feedback to the team
•responds in a problem-solving manner to the
   team's requests for help

pend on which phase of team development the ongoing member is in and also on the attitude of the ongoing member toward the team.

In addition to knowledge of their own profession, providers on an IHCT should have an understanding of the knowledge and roles of other team members. This understanding develops interprofessional trust and a willingness to share patients. Although the collective expertise of the practitioners on an IHCT should address the complex needs of patients, the planned structuring of this collective expertise is very difficult. Unlike therapy, encounter, and task groups where membership can be carefully planned, IHCT membership is subject to shifts in organizational priorities, often the result of changes or cutbacks in external funding. An IHCT's membership is also affected by two phenomena that are common in health settings (i.e., a high rate of staff turnover and the practice of rotating staff.)[4] At times, the membership of an IHCT might not reflect any well-conceived plan and the combined knowledge of the professionals assigned could be insufficient to meet either the team or patient needs. It is therefore important for a team to periodically monitor its personal and professional expertise and to match them to the needs of the patients who are served by the team.

Intra-team Components: Structure and Process

Initial development and continued training are part of the team's internal structure and process. Developing and maintaining the intra-team components of the IHCT can help members understand differences in individual and professional characteristics and ultimately should improve the team's output. Intra team components reflect both the needs of its patients and the survival needs of the team. The issue of trust is central to the development of the team. It involves knowledge of role performance (i.e., consistency of action—"I trust you because I know that you will do what you are supposed to do"). The affective component of trust involves emotional bonds between members. These are based on developing a consistency of action that involves structures and processes.

Establishing the internal structure of the team is one of the first tasks for a new team. Internal structure might include team mission, goals, protocols for patient care, kinds of meetings that will be held, who will formally lead, expected roles, and mechanisms that will be used for informal communication. Health professionals have a love–hate relationship with meetings. Some think of them as the bane of their existence and others think of them as necessary. Formal meetings are only one tool for communication and sharing information. Informal meetings and telephone conversations are more common and perhaps more important tools for team communication.

E-mail, voice mail, and progress notes are additional means of information sharing but are not good forms of communication as they do not permit interactive dialogue. As part of a team's structure, policies for using these tools should be written and adapted to the needs of the team.

Team structure usually is more static than team process and therefore is easier for new members to learn. However, even team structures must continually adapt to changes in the organizational environment. As the team develops, it should continually assure that its structures for problem solving and recording promote team dialogue. Left to their own devices, there is a strong tendency for health professionals to retreat to their discipline specific modes for setting, solving, and recording complex problems. When charts are sectioned by discipline, it is a good indication that the team is not interdisciplinary. The structure of patient treatment plans and assessment protocols can help prevent this from happening. The treatment plan should be a unified and dynamic document to which all disciplines relate. Problems should be written globally as interdisciplinary problems to which relevant disciplines can connect. An interdisciplinary problem encompasses those issues preventing a patient from achieving maximum independence. Progress notes should relate to the interdisciplinary treatment plan and all team members should write in the same section of the chart.

Team process and structure are interactive. For example, team process can be facilitated or hindered by strategically placing the desks of professionals from different disciplines. Placing team members' offices on different floors or in different buildings can strain efficient team communication. Structuring specific times to be on a particular unit is a formal way to enhance informal communication. New team members can be placed in close proximity to established members to both hasten and shape orientation. Team members taking an active role in program improvement can quickly alter team structure to meet the team's needs.

Establishing formal and informal leadership within the team can alter the authority roles and power structures of different professionals. A team physician may have higher authority than a nurse or social worker in terms of clinical decision making, but the nurse or social worker might be the formal team leader. Either leader can have a profound influence on how the team makes clinical decisions. A physician, social worker, nurse, or occupational therapist will assume leadership roles, as their professional or personal skills are needed in specific situations.

A team adopts processes for accomplishing its work and over time these processes become norms, a part of the team's unwritten structure. A team's norms may include how decisions are made, leadership is carried out, and conflict is managed. Norms can address either task or socioemotional issues. Procedures and roles develop as unquestioned norms early in a team's development. Cultural norms that define a team's values and collective beliefs usually take longer to form. However, it is quite possible for several powerful team members to share cultural norms and thus speed up the assimilation of those norms into the team's work. For example, team members who came from a teaching background might all apply the cultural norm of teaching and learning to the team. That team will develop with that norm until enough new members without that norm enter the team and overtly or covertly challenge the norm. That prompts the team to work on the process of re-affirming or changing the norm. As a team develops, its cultural norms (good and bad) gain strength and become more resistant to change. For this reason, it is good team practice for members to periodically identify and question a team's unwritten rules.

Informal and formal roles and tasks are negotiated around the team's goals. The initial goal setting and planning for patient care activities, record keeping, and administrative activities are at the heart of team decision making. New team members should be taught the informal and formal roles of team members and should be invited to openly question those roles. Ideally, team members will periodically examine the process factors that promote or hinder their interdependent problem solving.

Organizational Components: Internal and External

It is difficult for an IHCT to grow without having established effective relations with its organizational environment. Unlike a task group that is structured to accomplish a specific task within a defined time period, an IHCT survives over time by managing its resources within the confines of current market and political conditions. The team can strengthen its leadership position in the organization by periodically engaging in systems analysis and environmental scanning to recognize differences between its culture and the organization's culture. The rules of the broader external organization—congressional mandates or a changing mission in the chief executive's office—can be applied to teams in rigid or flexible ways. It is imperative that team members interact with the administration via committee membership, informal communication, and through formal administrative channels to monitor changing organizational climates. This organizational component is often left out of IHCT curricula, yet it is one of the most important variables for a team's survival. When teams do not form and sustain relations with the organization there is a danger of developing a "we" versus "they" attitude. If such a situation develops, the team will usually suffer.

There are many and emerging organizational structures that can support IHCTs. However, IHCTs in health care organizations are often structured as matrix systems. The members of the team may be hired and have their performance appraisals written by the director of their professional department, hopefully with input from a member(s) of the team. Team members must therefore learn to strike some balance between their professional department and their IHCT. The IHCT generally becomes stronger when the balance is in favor of the team.

Organizations may need to intervene in situations where there is a power struggle between the team and a department head. For example, if a department head continually schedules departmental meetings during the only time that the team has to meet, the problem needs to be addressed, either by the team member from that discipline or by someone higher in the team's administrative structure.

Components Necessary for Team Maintenance Over Time

Team maintenance is the fourth major part of the IHCT model and its central focus is functional or informal leadership, not necessarily linked to any management position. Anderson and Gevitz[5] described the team approach in general hospitals as one in which no member takes on total responsibility. However, for an IHCT to survive over time, every team member must assume some responsibility for team maintenance. If the IHCT is a self-managing team, all of its members should be expected to assume leadership functions. This leadership may be different from the formal leadership that is part of the structural component of the team (i.e., this leadership is different from the position of team manager).

Functional or informal leadership relates to the ability of each team member to take on leadership roles as team tasks call for their expertise. It is leadership that is assumed by the member of the team who is the most competent to assume it in a given situation. This concept of informal leadership refers to members' obligations to monitor and question how individual practice components, intrateam components, and broader organizational components promote the team's goals. When team members assume informal leadership they assume power for decision making in regard to change.

To maintain its capacity for interdependent collaborative decisions and to survive over time it is imperative that the team performs its maintenance functions. This team maintenance variable addresses the ability of all members to use power for dissent and decision making. On a developed team, each member has power for decision making, although member power is not necessarily equal because each member has a different body of knowledge and varied experience. Attention to this area can direct the team toward collaboration and innovation. The paradox and central assumption in this IHCT model is that the team (not individual members) controls the power for its internal decision making. However, the team cannot control the power for decision making unless every member takes some responsibility for informal leadership. The assumption is that a mature IHCT has developed sufficiently so that control of decision-making power is not held by only one or two members and the sense of having power for decision making is perceived by every member. A functioning IHCT can take many forms and have a variable mix of professionals, but is not well developed until it promotes the engagement of all members in interdependent collaboration.

EVOLUTION OF THE TEAM AND ITS MEMBERS

The four components of IHCTs and their variables not only interact with one another, but they also relate to the five phases of development and decision making: *forming, norming, confronting, performing*, and *leaving*. Each phase focuses on particular tasks and behaviors as it emphasizes different variables within the team model. Members may be in different phases from other team members, focusing on different team issues. The three main recurring phases are norming, confronting, and performing. The forming and leaving phases are in the model because they have significant, albeit intermittent, impact on a continuing IHCT. Because of the urgency of the work in health care settings, the initial forming phase can be very transitional. With reference to the leaving phase, the entire team seldom dissolves. These two phases have more relevance to individual members who enter or leave an existing IHCT but can also have profound effects on the team. The rate of staff turnover is an important variable in the development and maintenance of any organization. However, the reactions that continuing members have to a leaving member and the eventual introduction of a replacement dictate the importance of these two phases to any given team. The recurring influence of the leaving phase is the potential to advance or return the team to one of the other recurring phases.

The *team phase* represents the phase of the majority of members. However, it is common for individual members to perceive themselves in a developmental phase that differs from that of the collective team. New team members might influence the entire team or some of its members to revert to a less advanced phase. Also, members experiencing changes in their personal or professional lives might alter their commitment to the team and regress in relation to the team's phase. Lack of staff can prompt supervisors to assign team members from other areas of the organization to the team. Often these team members are assigned to the team for low percentages of time. This limited commitment may impede a member's progression to more advanced phases of development in relation to the team. Members with less than full-time commitments to the team might have difficulty keying in to the developmental phase of the entire team. The influence that part-time and transient members have on the further development of a well-functioning team is unclear and is likely dependent on personal and professional factors that they possess. When members leave the team, informal leadership shifts. A new member might be expected to assume a leadership role based on performance of a prior member from the same professional discipline. Assuming a key leadership role can prompt even a new member to move quickly to a more advanced phase of team development.[6] It is important for administrators and team leaders to realize that the stalled development of an IHCT might be the result of limited resources to address the team's work, lack of guidance in team development, or limited time to address process or structural issues. Table 2.2 depicts the phases of IHCT development and also addresses some interventions to help achieve the tasks necessary to move through or maintain each phase.

Forming Phase

Members of IHCTs are usually rushed to form a team and to begin performing their duties from their discipline's perspective. Instead of establishing team goals and roles or identifying personal and professional attributes that might help a team form or work through inevitable conflicts, an IHCT will likely repress the conflict and charge into the norming phase. Team members who are new to an existing IHCT go through the forming phase at various rates. The rates depend on the amount and quality of their prior team experience, how quickly they engage with a group, how actively they want to learn the ways of the team, and how quickly the other team members expect them to assume a given role. If the IHCT has already developed an early culture of "getting to work and ignoring conflict," the newer team members will likely act in the same manner.

Norming Phase

In groups, the second phase of development is the conflict or storming phase. Health care professionals generally do not wish to or are not given the time to work through their conflicts. They are expected to get to work. Thus, in this model the first recurring phase is norming. This direct move into norming interferes with questioning and might place the team in a

Table 2.2
Developmental Phases of Interdisciplinary Health Care Teams: Symptoms and Interventions

Phase I: Forming

Symptoms	Interventions
Superficially share name and background information	Create icebreakers (potlucks, informal discussions)
Members size up and test each other; categorize by professional roles and status	Discuss formal and potential informal roles of members; verbalize stated team goals
Members guarded, more impersonal than personal, some active, most passive	Encourage informal time to get to know one another
Uncertain about team membership	New team--discuss and agree on core and secondary team membership. New team member--mentor should discuss and assure understanding
Conflict is neither discussed nor addressed	Encourage conflict recognition as an opportunity for creative problem solving

Phase II: Norming

Symptoms	Interventions
Difficult to understand goals and purpose of the team	Discuss the goals as a team

continued

Attempt to establish common team goals	Discuss and agree as a team
Mistrust each other; exhibit caution and conformity	Structure opportunities for informal communication about training, values, experience, and duties of each member
Begin to see role overlaps	Observe members from other disciplines; discuss overlaps
Know conflicts are present; cover them up or whitewash them	Encourage conflict recognition as an opportunity for creative problem solving
A few members attempt to establish bonds with others who have similar views	Form a subcommittee and include members from different coalitions
Team establishes ground rules; begins to clarify common roles	Reinforce ground rules; negotiate common roles
Team may want leader(s) to assume responsibility	Identify informal leadership roles that need to be filled and who can fill them
Team tries strategies to increase equality of leadership (e.g., rotating leaders)	Emphasize development of competence for different leadership roles
Defensive communication and disruptive behavior increases	At process team meeting, give open feedback and discuss patterns of disruption and solutions

continued

Symptoms	Interventions
Team members are frustrated	Promote informal leadership for resolving problems
Some members project blame and responsibility toward the perceived leaders	Promote informal leadership for resolving problems
Team members compete	Discuss different leadership roles; praise members for individual contributions
Some members come to meetings late or do not attend them	Review rules for membership (e.g., attendance at meetings, start and end meetings on time, ignore late arrivals)

Phase III: Confronting

Symptoms	Interventions
Can no longer avoid conflicts; some members verbally attack other members	Bring team conflicts to team forum or process leader (if identified); process leader mediates between individuals
Conflicts of leadership, equality, commitment increase	Identify, clarify, and assign informal leadership roles
Members feel anxiety over expression of affect	Encourage expressions of affect–positive and negative
Address some conflicts directly	Encourage the practice of constructive confrontation; focus on solutions to problems

continued

Symptoms	Interventions
Some members withdraw from the team	Review reasons for leaving; may be a symptom of team dysfunction
Search for leader who will resolve conflicts	Identify members with skills and willingness to assume role of process analyzer
Functional leaders emerge	Identify and encourage informal leaders
Realize that power is not equal	Identify all potential power sources
Realize that everyone has power for leadership and decision making	Encourage members to recognize and assume power sources they are capable of assuming
Conflicts lead to constructive confrontation	Help the team (members) discuss and resolve conflicts; regard as opportunity for creative problem solving
Team reclarifies goals and roles	As a team, update goals; discuss roles and agree
Form coalitions that change according to needs of the team	Praise this as sign of team's growth

Phase IV: Performing

Symptoms	Interventions
Appreciate differences of members	Encourage this behavior

23

continued

Members encourage and help each other	Identify and encourage as team's culture
Increase reality testing; team grows stronger	Schedule open feedback of members to team
The norm is self-initiated active participation	Praise informal leadership
Members trust each other and develop strong relationships	Enjoy; offer to mentor new members
Members meet regularly and come on time	Reinforce as part of team culture
See conflicts as normal and use as impetus for program improvement	Reinforce as part of team culture
Emphasize productivity and problem solving	Reinforce as part of team culture
Members responsible for leadership in teaching, wherever skills warrant it	Reinforce as part of team culture; assure all informal leadership roles are filled

Phase V: Leaving
individual leaves

Symptoms	Interventions
Individual feels anger toward members or the team in general	Praise the member for team accomplishments; wish members well in new endeavor

continued

Members deny impending departure because of disbelief and regret	As a team, discuss interim situation; plan for replacement
Team expresses wish for member to remain with the team	Accept as a sign of a significant loss to team; regard as potential ghost for team to address in the future
Team may regress to an earlier phase	Determine the team's developmental phase; proceed from there
Individual may express happiness over leaving the team	Accept that the member is happy and that the team has a shortage to address

team terminates

Symptoms	Interventions
Some members withdraw; depression and sadness result	Develop a team plan of action; develop a personal plan of action
Members express team's superiority	Celebrate and record the team's accomplishments
Express feelings as testimonials	Listen and encourage team members to express their feelings and plan for their future
Affirm team membership as a valuable experience	Celebrate with an eye to the future

groupthink mentality. Conflict is usually kept under the table in the norming phase. This causes frustration to build as this phase progresses and, rather than addressing the team problems, members have a tendency to retreat into their comfortable discipline-specific ways of operating. It is common for health care teams to become stuck in this phase. Many IHCTs never progress beyond norming because health care practitioners do not like conflict and use many excuses for ignoring it. If the team encounters a lot of change and does not address conflicts it is continually recycled back into the early norming phase.

As the norming phase progresses, it is common for IHCTs to strive for equality of leadership. Teams may initiate rotating leadership for various tasks, irrespective of the qualifications and constraints of individual members. The team might ignore the fact that the pharmacist does not have the skills or desire to run the team meeting or that the physician does not have the time to do the preparatory work. The team expects them to take turns with the rest of the team's members. Competition between disciplines might also occur based on expectations of equality. Because there is role overlap between health professions, members from different disciplines might vie to interview a particular patient, insist on being the first to see a patient in clinic, question whether it is the social worker's role to call a nursing director, or question whether it is the nurse's role to check on a placement for a patient. The conflict becomes more difficult to keep under the table as the team approaches the confronting phase.

Confronting Phase

Conflict erupts and is addressed in the confronting phase. The early part of this phase can be quite uncomfortable for the team. The emergence of conflict might frighten some members who move back to the overtly more comfortable norming phase where conflict is usually covered up. In the confronting phase, members realize the power of constructive confrontation and use the opportunity to engage in problem solving behavior. As informal leaders emerge there is a realization that, although every member must have power for decision making, the power is not equal. As members realize their potential for power it enables the assumption of informal leadership roles for the team.

The IHCT begins to move into the performing phase when individual members demonstrate their power in the process of collaboration. Members might also protect the rights of their fellow members to use power. By establishing the right to individual power as a norm, the team assures that a few members do not assume all of the power and that every member has power for decision making. When this occurs, constructive confrontation becomes a team norm. The initial team goals and roles should be re-examined (perhaps with heated debate) in this phase. Re-examining goals and roles may involve an increase in disruptive behavior. The team's approach to the inevitable conflict depends on its maturity level and the conflict and decision-making styles of the team's members. Each time this occurs, the team builds on prior history and re-establishes itself with more depth and maturity.

Performing Phase

The team is performing when the conflicts are directed more at program development than at individual members. Also, the differences of each team member become an appreciated addition to the team. Members trust each other enough to view conflicts as normal and essential to further team development. This tends to be a phase that teams visit occasionally. When there are constant and intense changes in a health care system IHCTs will not remain in this phase for long periods.

Leaving Phase

The leaving phase may not be included in some team models. Although this phase is intermittent, it is an important part of a team's development because it is normal for IHCTs to have some turnover. Leaving might be temporary or permanent, might involve one or many members, and some of those members will be powerful team leaders and some will be members with limited capacity for team function. The qualities of the leaving members will be reflected in how much the team grieves or denies the changes that take place as the member exits. Occasionally, the entire team can be threatened with termination as an organization chooses to downsize. In such cases, there can be a powerful effect on the entire organization as the team's members choose different methods to cope with their loss.

Both the ongoing team members and the entire team might continue to recycle through any of the phases of team development as they encounter personal or professional problems or as the team encounters change.

MOVEMENT THROUGH THE PHASES

This team development model is complex and dynamic. In imagining the way a team and its members move through the phases of development, it might be helpful to think of an IHCT as a flattened sphere, much like a large ball of rigid plastic material. Team members circle this ball as they attempt

Figure 2.1
Emerging Interdisciplinary Health Care Team in the Norming Phase

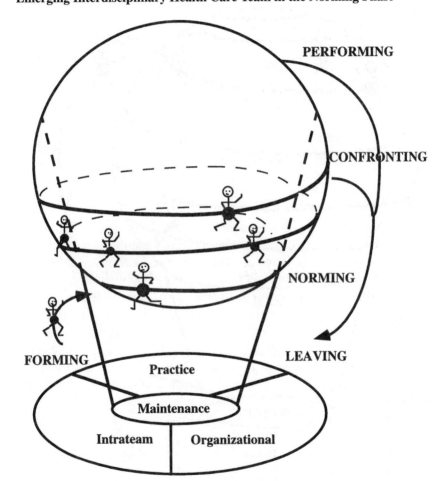

Figure 2.2
Ongoing Poorly Developed Health Care Team Struggling to Survive

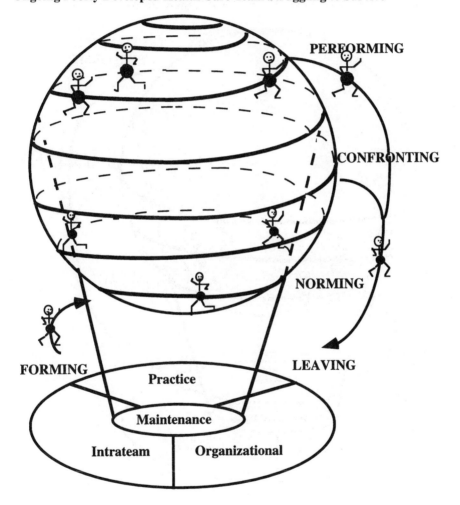

Figure 2.3
Well-Functioning Interdisciplinary Health Care Team

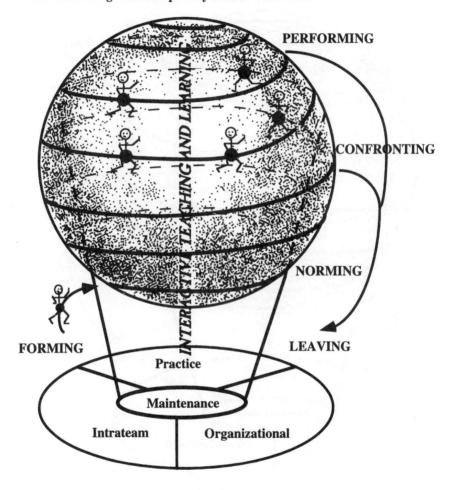

Figure 2.4
Interdisciplinary Health Care Team in Chaos

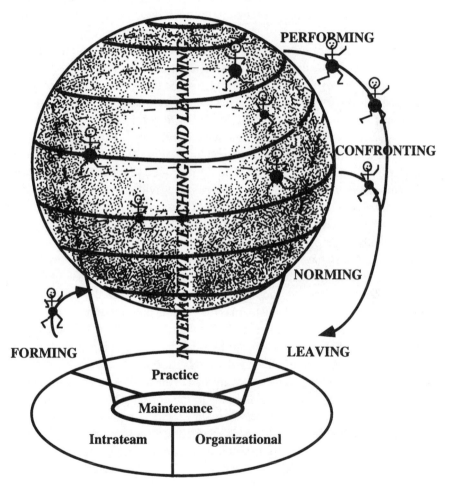

to make the team functionally responsive to the tasks at hand. In a deflated condition, this ball will only roll one way. However, as the ball inflates (representing a team with a developing culture) it rolls more freely and can roll in any direction as problems dictate. As the team develops toward the performing phase and concurrently develops its culture, the team becomes three dimensional. The foundation for a team is the set of components and variables (practice, intrateam, organizational, and maintenance) that are essential to its function. The interdisciplinary teaching and learning is the channel through which the team maintains itself by assuring that its components are working together. The closer the team gets to its ideal condition (the inflated ball), the more it can gauge the content, context, and timing for the teaching and learning to occur. Also, the closer the team is to its ideal condition the more time it generally takes for the team to return to a compromised condition. In other words, as the team develops its culture it is able to withstand setbacks while retaining its ability to solve complex problems.

Tables 2.1 and 2.2 are complementary to Figures 2.1 through 2.4. The stick people in the figures represent team members as they proceed through the phases of team development. The figures depict numerous features of this team development model (e.g., team vs. individual development), differing developmental phases, direction of movement, rate of movement, newer versus longer term team members, and flatness (Figures 2.1 and 2.2) versus depth (Figures 2.3 and 2.4) of team culture.

Individual team members do not always join a team at the same time. Because of this, some members find themselves in a different phase of development from the rest of the team. Another reason for this differential development of individual and team is the varying amount of time that some members are assigned to the team. Full-time team members might engage more rapidly with the team. Some individuals are more likely than others to enjoy working on a team. Other individuals might just take a long time to trust others. And, individuals who were sent to the team against their desires may never progress beyond the forming or the norming phases. It is important for team members to watch for other members who are having difficulty assimilating into the team so they can offer support and possible assistance. Teams, especially long-term ones, may have some members in each phase of team development as in Figure 2.4. This makes it difficult to determine the true phase of the team. A team in this situation is probably in chaos and members should use this chaos as an indication that they need to engage in some formal team development.

Team members can proceed in different directions and at different rates through the model, dependent on changing practice and intrateam and organizational factors. The team components and phases of development as depicted in Tables 2.1 and 2.2 are the influences that spark successes or failures in the team. Each member of the team can recognize or ignore the ever-changing team components in Table 2.1. Each member can view these team components as either positive or negative stresses. The prevalent perceptions draw individual members and the entire team either up toward performing as in Figure 2.3 or down toward norming as in Figure 2.1.

Each stick person represents the phase of a member. The phase that contains the majority of stick figures is the current phase of the team (e.g., the team in Figure 2.1 is in the norming phase because four of the team's six members are in the norming phase). The larger stick figures represent team members who have been with the team for more than a year and the smaller stick figures represent members who have been with the team for less than a year. A larger stick person in the forming or norming phase as in Figure 2.1 would indicate a member who may be working within their discipline, but who is not engaged with the team. A smaller stick person in the confronting or performing phase as in Figure 2.4 would indicate a member who quickly engaged with the team and moved through the phases. It is likely someone who was trained to work on an IHCT or someone who has worked on IHCTs in the past.

This model is dynamic in that it reflects the growing depth and resilience of an established team. A newly forming IHCT, without a sense of history, would be depicted as a unidimensional flat entity as in Figure 2.1. In this team all of the stick people are in either the forming or the norming phases (although one member is approaching the confronting phase). Team members have not yet begun to confront team conflicts. Figure 2.2 represents an ongoing IHCT that has some longer term members. Some members who are performing in relation to the team are likely informal leaders. However, the team is still a flat entity as it has not begun to address its conflicts, and although some members are in the performing phase the team has no cultural depth. One longer term member is leaving (perhaps out of frustration) and newer members appear somewhat confused about their position in relation to the team.

An IHCT that has proceeded through the first three or four phases at least once takes on a multidimensional quality as in Figures 2.3 and 2.4. Such a team establishes a history and culture that helps it to re-examine new questions with a background of experience. If all members feel empowered to assume appropriate leadership, the team has the capacity to learn and grow using past mistakes to feed new ideas. The team represented in Figure 2.3 has a depth of culture that has come from working through its problems in an open and constructive manner. It is a healthy team moving toward performing. In contrast, the team in Figure 2.4 has probably experienced major recent changes. As stated earlier, it is a team in chaos. However, because it has a depth of culture, it should be able to recognize its problems and develop strategies for addressing them. Depending on the extent of the change and the loss of the team's leaders, it might temporarily move to the norming phase before it recovers.

IHCTs may not always follow a specific order of development or development may occur so quickly that the sequence is imperceptible. After forming, IHCTs may quickly establish norms because they are under pressure to perform. However these initial norms often promote discipline specific goals and do not insure good outcomes for complex problems. Some IHCTs might remain in a static state of norming for long periods of time. On the other hand, an IHCT might proceed directly from norming to performing, especially when its members are experienced at working with other disciplines. It is probable that such a team has not been challenged by conflict, and even though well functioning it does not possess the depth of culture to survive over time. Additionally, it is common for newer teams to view themselves as performing when it is clear that they avoid the constructive use of conflict and have little depth of culture. The current phase of the IHCT may not denote the depth of the team's development because a well-developed team may temporarily revert to the *norming* phase. However, with leaders who are in more advanced phases, it should quickly recover and increase its depth.

A Case of Miscommunication or of Poor Team Function?

A social worker on a clinical outreach team with several nurses discovered that a patient of hers had fallen the previous day. The nurse, the only team member to be alerted, had found someone to stay with the patient, but had not informed the social worker of this. This effort had taken the nurse many hours and because she also had nursing visits to make she ended up working until 9 p.m. In speaking with the patient about placement in a group home, the nurse discovered that the patient wanted placement in a new group home that was near her home. The nurse promised the patient that she would try to place her in that home and called to begin the arrangements. She found that the outreach program did not have a contract with the new home for payment and also had no information on the quality of the home.

The social worker for the clinical outreach team was not contacted until late the next morning when the nurse asked about using the new group home. The social worker told the nurse of the difficulty and the nurse continued to stress how important it was for this patient to be close to her home and that the patient was really counting on it. The social worker told the nurse to ask their supervisor to make an exception and offered alternatives if the new group home did not work out. The supervisor refused the request and they placed the patient in an alternative home, which felt all right to the social worker because she anticipated that the patient would return home after 2 weeks. If the stay were to be permanent the so-cial worker would have tried harder but because it was a crisis she sensed that they should take what was available. The social worker felt that if she had been involved when the nurse became involved with the patient's fall, the place close to the pa-tient's home would never have been offered because the social worker knew that the agency had temporarily stopped establishing new providers. She could have helped prevent the nurse from working late by assisting with the planning.

Additionally, when the social worker talked to the daughter the day after the fall, the daughter said she felt bad that no one called her or her brother on the day of the fall. She was upset and her confidence in the program had been shaken. The daughter had requested to be called if something really serious happened to her mother. The social worker apologized that no one had called and assured her they would call in the future. The social worker knew that had she been informed earlier that she would have notified the daughter because it is easier for two people to think of all the important details. Also, the social worker considered contacting family members as an important part of her job.

It is interesting to speculate about the team in this case, what phase of de-velopment the team and its members might be in, and whether this team has any depth to its development. Some of the other issues to consider are whether this team has an interdisciplinary definition of the patient's prob-lems, what are the appropriate roles and tasks for nursing and social work, how team members might build more trust, and what other team-related problems might be related to the situation.

ACHIEVING EFFICIENCY: MATRIX OF
INTERDISCIPLINARY PROBLEM SOLVING

Efficiency involves time, resources, cost, and long-term outcomes. Health care organizations have traditionally measured short-term and fo-cused outcomes (e.g., length of visits, numbers of patients seen by each dis-cipline, or correctly dispensing a prescription). Longer term global health outcomes (which may represent a greater initial cost)—maintaining inde-pendent function, patient follow-through on treatment regimens, iatrogenic effects, and effects on family and caregivers—have often been ignored. Health care organizations continue to measure short-term focused out-comes because these organizations are based on a business production para-digm and are reimbursed for this type of outcome. Unfortunately, looking at short-term and focused outcomes usually does not work with complex and ambiguous problems.

If health care organizations have difficulty measuring long-term global outcomes, it is no wonder that they do not know how to measure the effi-

ciency of teamwork. Hiring team members and providing initial team training is not sufficient to ensure that a team will perform. In fact, if the
components of a team are in place and the team is well on its way toward the
performing phase it might still not be efficient in its problem solving. If
team members do not know which members to involve in discussions and
when to involve them, the team may unknowingly be using more resources
than it needs to use. To become efficient, the team must direct the interplay
between individual disciplines and the organization of the team as these relate to the types of problems team members encounter. Team members must
learn to define the scope of a problem in a way that is neither too narrow nor
too broad; identify the least disciplines needed to address the problem well;
and prioritize the assessments and interventions that are necessary to address the problem. Tables 2.3 and 2.4 might be useful for increasing the efficiency of interdisciplinary problem solving.

Table 2.3
Efficiency Estimates for Effects of Six Variables on Interdisciplinary
Intervention When a Problem Is Tame

	Appropriate Disciplines	Inappropriate Disciplines	
Greater Than One Discipline	Low	Low	Highly Organized
One Discipline	High	Low	Low Organization

Table 2.4
Efficiency Estimates for Effects of Six Variables on Interdisciplinary
Intervention When a Problem Is Wicked

	Appropriate Disciplines	Inappropriate Disciplines	
Greater Than One Discipline	High	Low	Highly Organized
One Discipline	Low	Low	Low Organization

Tame Versus Wicked Problems

Tame problems are those that can be defined. The outcome can be predicted and procedures for intervention can be quantified, measured, and replicated. Administering an influenza vaccination, diagnosing a simple cold or the stomach flu in a 10-year-old, treating an infected cut in a healthy person, and following up an uncomplicated gall bladder surgery are all relatively tame problems. They can and should be efficiently accomplished by one provider (see Table 2.3).

Wicked problems are on the opposite extreme. The term *wicked problem* was used by Rittel and Webber[7] and aptly captures the complexity and ambiguity that is inherent in many patient and team problems. In health care, a wicked problem is one that is difficult to formulate, has more than one explanation, is often a symptom of another problem, is frequently unique, and does not resolve with a simple intervention. Such a problem is multifaceted and many of those facets are intentionally or unintentionally hidden. The following are some examples of potentially wicked problems: scheduling an influenza vaccination in a demented elder who has had a prior adverse reaction to an influenza vaccine; treating a Cryptosporidium infection presenting as stomach flu and rheumatoid arthritis in a person recovering from cancer treatments; or treating an infected cut in a diabetic with poor vision who lives alone in a house with no running water. In order to achieve high efficiency, each of these cases will require input from more than one discipline (see Table 2.4).

There is a continuum that exists between wicked and tame problems and it is critical for practitioners to learn to accurately assess where on the continuum a problem lies. In the middle of the continuum lie moderate problems that may also call for more than one discipline. When the patient repeatedly returns with the same problem or when the patient is frail or in jeopardy, the problem moves further over to the wicked end of the scale. Assessing the type of problem is one of the most difficult aspects of interdisciplinary problem solving. It requires a realization by practitioners that one cannot solve the problem alone. It also requires open dialogue with members of more than one discipline. A clinician who is taught autonomous practice will look at the presenting problem through discipline specific glasses and ignore others. Consequently, the clinician can miss the significance of a wicked problem and might ignore the potential for other disciplines to help solve the problem. In the interest of team efficiency, practitioners must be taught how to recognize and treat both tame and wicked problems.

Words of Advice

How an IHCT assesses and treats a wicked problem is a good indicator of the depth of the team's interdisciplinary culture and of the efficiency and effectiveness of the team.

Using Appropriate Disciplines

Whether the problem is tame or wicked, having the appropriate team members address it is a key to attaining efficiency on an IHCT. If the problem is tame and one person can handle it, that person should be the team member who is most expert in that particular area. This requires that team members know their own competencies and have an awareness of the core knowledge base of other disciplines. It also entails knowing how different disciplines frame problems and problem solve. For example, faced with a brittle case of juvenile diabetes, a physician might frame the problem as a need to titrate medication and monitor glucose levels. A nurse might frame the problem as a need for family education and ongoing monitoring. A social worker might frame the problem as one of educating peers and caregiver stress. There are obvious overlaps in the three ways of framing this problem because "monitoring" might involve patient, caregiver, and perhaps peers. Because this case of juvenile diabetes presents as a wicked problem it might take all three disciplines working together to frame the problem so that they can more efficiently resolve it.

How different disciplines are taught or not taught to work with practitioners from other disciplines is a major factor in whether they use the talents of other disciplines to help solve wicked problems. If practitioners from a certain discipline are taught to demonstrate an authoritarian leadership style it will be difficult for them to engage the willing services of other disciplines. If practitioners from another discipline are always expected to defer to other more highly trained practitioners it will hinder their willingness to offer constructive ideas for care. If practitioners from a given discipline are taught to "do their own thing" without taking into account the input of other practitioners, that is what they will do. All of this affects the economics of team practice.

Every discipline has areas of overlap with other disciplines. Practitioners frequently take advantage of areas of overlap by assuming duties that might be considered more in the domain of another profession. For example, a general medical nurse or an occupational therapist might attempt some assessment and intervention of a patient's depression. For mild cases, this will work fine. However, if the patient's depression is complicated by a long-standing personality disorder or occasional manic episodes, the clinician may be in over his or her head without realizing it. The clinicians in this case should know the core competencies of psychiatry, psychology, and social work and should call in the appropriate discipline(s). The patient's problems might best respond to a plan by the occupational therapist, social worker, and psychiatrist. In this case, the nurse would bow out for the time being.

A busy nurse who has some skill in identifying resources to support a patient in the community may be out of his or her league when those resources depend on uncertain funding sources, an area in which the social worker is current. A social worker who realizes that a family is living on junk food might speak with family members about their eating habits, but if the problem is serious a dietitian could counsel the family more efficiently and with greater impact. These examples point out the value of understanding the skills of other disciplines that enable the practitioner to call in a more appropriate practitioner before a situation consumes limited resources.

It is also important for practitioners to learn the difference between professional competencies and other learned competencies that team members might have. A nursing assistant might be good at listening to a patient's problems and at giving that patient sound advice. When that nursing assistant leaves and is replaced by another, it would be common for members of other disciplines to expect the replacement to have the same counseling skills as the previous nursing assistant when, in fact, it is not one of the job skills for that position. There is also a difference between competencies and personalities. For example, team members might expect that all social workers will project a sense of protecting the self-determination of the patient or that all nurses will exhibit very caring behavior toward patients. Although some of these behaviors are built into each profession, there is wide latitude in behaviors that are exercised by virtue of different personalities.

Knowing the core competencies of different disciplines and the levels within each discipline is critical not only for members of IHCTs, but also for health care administrators. In order to hire and or engage the correct disciplines, an administrator must know what each discipline is expected to do well. An administrator will need this knowledge to communicate with internal and external funding sources about the needs of the patients and the best way to meet those needs.

There are gray areas of discipline knowledge, areas that individuals trained in a particular discipline know something about but are not expert in. Physicians as a profession used to dwell in those gray areas. In recent years, that role has been assumed by nurses. With cost containment and limited funding for dealing with wicked problems, the discipline that takes responsibility for coordination and integration (nursing) has taken over the gray areas of health care. Administrators have accepted nursing in these roles because it leads them to believe that they can eliminate other disciplines and reap cost savings by doing so. However, no one discipline can do every thing well and efficiently, especially when dealing with wicked problems. Accepting a discipline as a universal provider confuses other disciplines and can also confuse the discipline that is accepting that role. The intent here is to raise this issue as something that has the potential to affect any discipline and that can interfere with the effectiveness and efficiency of patient care and interdisciplinary practice.

Calling in another discipline when there is a wicked problem in a gray area requires more than consulting with that discipline. If the problem is a wicked one it will require a dialogue and joint action between individuals from several disciplines. To achieve maximum efficiency, there will need to be a system of identifying such problems so that a variety of disciplines can relate to them. Additionally, the team needs a mechanism for identifying the presenting problem and allied problems in relation to an integrated goal (i.e., frame it as an interdisciplinary problem). The team can then create stepped-in procedures for different disciplines to move in and out of the maze as it moves the patient toward long-term resolution.

Level of Team Organization Required

The efficiency of an IHCT hinges on defragmenting the structure and processes involved in the assessment and care plan. One of the early tasks of an IHCT should be to structure a unified assessment and treatment process. This activity will have a profound impact on the development of a new IHCT. It forces members to discuss what their discipline specific roles are and what their roles will be in relation to the team. Continuing its development a team should move on to discussing and adapting its standards of practice and critical pathways for common and recurring patient problems. If this is done in the context of the team's unified assessment and treatment structure and process, the team will be well on its way to performing and delivering excellent care. The IHCT needs to develop and maintain the structure of a unified assessment or treatment process. Likewise, it needs to establish one place for charting progress notes related to the interdisciplinary treatment plan.

Organizing the team's meeting structure and process are also part of the efficiency of teams. Staff will either model or avoid the types of meetings that they have been exposed to in the past. If meetings are ill planned, begin late, and have little focus, busy providers will learn to avoid them at all costs. On the other hand, if team members experience well-run interdisciplinary meetings that start and end on time, involve the right mix of disciplines, are run by a qualified meeting leader, are focused, and encourage dialogue on relevant new knowledge, they will model those types of meetings within and across team boundaries.

An IHCT needs protocols and procedures for members to act, react, and interact with each other on a continuous basis, not just at weekly staff meetings. Framing and expressing problems, not as discreet entities but as pieces of an integrated whole are essential aspects of the efficient IHCT.

Just because numerous disciplines are relevant to a wicked problem does not mean that they all have to physically evaluate the patient. In an IHCT that is highly organized, one or two disciplines might be responsible for conducting an initial assessment. Some of the disciplines would be advising a smaller core team on how to handle the problem. Questioning and teaching would flow freely across disciplines. In the case of a family living on junk food the dietitian might just advise the social worker until the social worker established enough trust so that the family would agree to interact directly with the dietitian.

Words of Advice

Interdisciplinary health care teams must be highly organized entities. If an IHCT is not organized and functional there is no possibility that its full talents can be used when needed.

Every practitioner encounters situations on a daily basis that require intervention by one discipline. Practitioners also encounter situations that require a highly organized team. If the resources of an entire team are used to engage tame problems, it is not an efficient use of resources and is seen by practitioners as a waste of time (see Table 2.3). On the other hand, if no team is available to address wicked problems, it is not only inefficient (see Table 2.4), but can be very costly and frustrating for the practitioner and the patient. Learning to distinguish the type of structure needed for a given situation is a skill that must be acquired by practitioners. Learning how much and what kinds of structures are needed to address different types of problems are critical skills for an IHCT.

Paradox of Interdisciplinary Thinking

Interdisciplinary thinking involves the maximum amount of autonomy with the least amount of anarchy (turmoil). Turmoil can come from the patient, the family, the system, co-workers, other disciplines, the team, and from within yourself.

METHODS OF TEAM PRACTICE

Some practitioners erroneously believe that being a member of an IHCT means that they must give up autonomous practice or conversely that most decisions should be brought to the team. Although most health care practice is autonomous, health professionals must also be able to recognize when a complex situation calls for input from members of their own or other disciplines. In fact, autonomous practice is one of at least six methods of team practice, that is, *autonomous*; the *ad hoc group* or *task group*, which meets to work on a specific issue and then disbands; the *formal work group* that is ongoing and consists of professionals from one discipline; the *formal work group* of many disciplines; the *one-discipline interactive team* that works on its developmental processes; and the *interactive team* that is interdisciplinary. A family practitioner working regularly with a gastroenterologist and a psychiatrist serving patients with eating disorders would be using a unidisciplinary method of practice because they are all physicians and have formalized their process. If they provide information to one another and each make independent decisions they would be using a formal unidisciplinary work group method. If they are interdependent, openly discuss options, and reflect on their teamwork they are an interactive unidisciplinary team. If the family practitioner also works regularly with a clinical nurse specialist, social worker, and dietitian they would be using either multidisciplinary or interdisciplinary methods of team practice. If they provide information to one another and each make independent decisions, they would be using a formal multidisciplinary work group method. If they are interdependent, openly discuss options, and reflect on their teamwork, they are an interactive interdisciplinary team. If any or all of these professionals talked briefly together occasionally, informally, or both, they would be using an ad hoc task group method of teamwork. Each method of team practice has specific characteristics that are specified in Table 2.5.

There are advantages and disadvantages to each of the methods of team practice. The ad hoc group might be the appropriate method to rapidly address a unique problem with implications for the larger organization. However, because solutions of the ad hoc group often lack breadth and depth, it might not be an effective method for addressing complex ongoing practice issues. The multidisciplinary formal work group might be a good method for discussing routine health care that needs to involve input from many disciplines. However, because solutions from this method often lack depth, it is not an effective method for addressing complex issues that have no single solution and that tend to be ongoing.

When health care practitioners encounter a problem, whether patient-related or not, they have a decision to make. They can solve the problem alone or use one of the other forms of team practice. The choice of whether to contact someone else, who to contact and when, depends on their philosophy of practice, level of training, and security in opening themselves to another point of view. If a given situation calls for the skills of a single profession and a person from that profession feels comfortable applying those skills, he or she will likely work independently. If a situation is seen as demanding skills a professional does not have, he or she might consult another professional, either from the same or another discipline. The discipline that is chosen will depend on availability, potential of saving time, and the individual's knowledge of what that discipline has to offer. It will also involve some degree of trust, meaning that a professional needs to know something about the person he or she is contacting (i.e., knowledge base, values, methods of gathering and processing information, perceived accuracy, reliability, and speed of delivery). The practitioner might also assume, based on past experience or training, that a particular profession or department should be able to handle certain problems. This knowledge and past experience with another provider is the basis of trust and provides practitioners with the sense that their requests will be heeded.

If we do not know what other health care professionals know our expectations for them will be inaccurate. Credentials are not always sufficient as predictors of a practitioner's knowledge. Although it is essential to have an awareness of the expected knowledge base of the different levels within a profession, it is also very helpful to know how someone was trained. If we think we know what a health care professional should know (based only on their credentials) and ask someone of that profession for help on a case, then we may be dissatisfied with the results and will likely exclude that person from further dialogue. For example, we may think that a registered nurse should be able to suggest interventions for a patient who has a borderline personality disorder, cardiac insufficiency, chronic pain from rheumatoid arthritis, caregiver burden from caring for her demented spouse, and is not complying with her medications. If the registered nurse is a clinician with a master's degree, we would probably be correct in assuming that he or she could understand the issues. If the registered nurse has a 2-year nursing degree and little experience, we will likely be disappointed with the interaction and consequently may decide to tackle the problem ourselves, even though it could be done more efficiently with the help of a nurse. Alternately, we may choose to speak with a member of our own discipline because we have more trust in what to expect, even though this may be an inefficient use of our time. We may also waste time trying to contact a busy

Table 2.5
Methods of Interdisciplinary Health Care Practice

	Description
Ad Hoc/Task Group	≥ 1 discipline/department/agency Group selects or agrees on a leader Rules set by the group Solves a problem and disbands
Formal Unidisciplinary Work Group (e.g., MDs from multiple specialties)	One discipline/department/ ≥ 1 agency Members report to group Individual identities more important than integrated diagnoses Don't work on team problems Leadership by election or rank Discipline specific care
Formal Multidisciplinary Work Group (e.g., MD, RN, SW, OT)	> 1 discipline/department/ ≥ 1 agency Members report to group Individual identities more important than integrated diagnoses Don't work on team problems Leadership by election, or rank Discipline specific care
Interactive Unidisciplinary Team (e.g., MDs from multiple specialties)	One discipline/department/ ≥ 1 agency Integrated diagnoses Team goals for patient and team Members interdependent Team structures enable collaboration Work on team problems Leadership appropriate to issue/expertise
Interactive Interdisciplinary Team (e.g., MD, RN, SW, OT)	> 1 discipline/department/ ≥ 1 agency Integrated diagnoses Team goals for patient and team Members interdependent Team structures enable collaboration Work on team problems Leadership appropriate to issue/expertise
Autonomous Practice	Individual decides based on knowledge

Advantages	Disadvantages
Focus on one issue No elaborate rules Quick and dirty Members capture enthusiasm	Solutions lack depth/breadth Some fear expressing views Status may hinder openness Difficulty getting together
Members speak same language Final decisions by formal leader Ongoing Rules established to keep order Security of one discipline Solutions may have depth	Some resent leaders decisions Solutions lack breadth May miss important problems Little integrative dialogue Inefficient with complexity
Final decisions by formal leader Ongoing Rules established to keep order Information from many perspectives Solutions may have breadth	Some resent leaders decisions Speak different languages Solutions not integrated Different cultures of disciplines not used advantageously Little integrative dialogue Inefficient with complexity

Members speak same language
Share responsibility for leadership
More openness
More informal collaboration
Solutions have depth
Members feel empowered
Culture encourages creativity
	Initial decisions take more time
	Solutions may lack breadth
	May miss important problems
	Need time and space to discuss
	  values; renegotiate roles,
	  leadership, conflict

Integrated care
Share responsibility for leadership
Solutions address complex problems
Solutions have depth and breadth
Members feel empowered
Creative approaches to complexity
Understand autonomous practice
	Initial decisions take more time
	Members must learn different
	  languages/terms
	Effort to maintain the team
	Need time and space to clarify
	  values; renegotiate roles,
	  leadership, conflict

Quick, appropriate solutions	Works only if understands interdisciplinary practice

physician when we could have more efficiently asked an appropriately trained and lesser paid nurse. We might also have asked a clinical pharmacist. These are typical decisions of everyday practice for all health care practitioners. And yet, we are seldom taught to make these choices. Instead, we are taught to function in the "safe" world of our own narrow practice range.

Although health professionals recognize the need to interact with others in the health care community, it is difficult for them to do so unless they have received training in all six methods of teamwork. Health care practitioners cannot choose the most appropriate type of practice if they are not familiar and comfortable with their options. The six methods of team practice need to be mastered if a practitioner is to be efficient and effective. Knowing how to use one method of team practice does not assure knowing how to use another (e.g., if one knows how to work in an ad hoc task group one does not necessarily know how to work in a multidisciplinary team). Learning to use the six methods of team practice is not necessarily progressive. Learning the autonomous practice of one's own discipline also does not have to precede learning about each of the other methods of team practice. At every level of training, it is necessary for health care practitioners to learn the skills of interdisciplinary practice and the types of interaction necessary for different levels of patient problems. Learning to operate as a member of an IHCT is the only way to assure knowledge of all of the other methods of team practice. Although time intensive, there is an efficiency in training for interdisciplinary practice. Figure 2.5 illustrates this point. As individual practitioners and teams learn about the six methods of team practice and the most appropriate method for a given problem, they gain depth and breadth in their ability to problem solve. Both the team's members and the team become able to address increasingly complex issues. The efficiency of teamwork is achieved by correctly matching team method with the situation.

A Paradox of Good Health Care

To appropriately choose autonomous practice, a health practitioner must have a working knowledge of what other disciplines do and a knowledge of how an interactive team operates.

MATCHING PROBLEM AND PRACTICE METHOD

Thinking of the IHCT as a fluid system of practice helps make it more understandable. In learning efficiency within the system of interdisciplinary practice, all methods of team practice should be part of the arsenal of the health care professional. The need for ongoing interdependence and collab-

Figure 2.5
Interdisciplinary Teamwork System

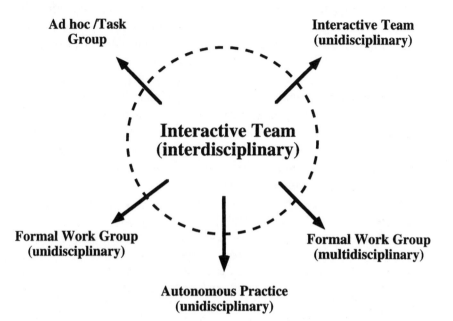

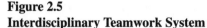

oration are triggers to which method of team practice is right to address a problem, whether it is related to patient care or system operation. If an IHCT is to function well and be accepted as part of its broader organizational structure it must also have the capacity to adapt to changing and complex situations.

IHCTs provide structure that enables health professionals to work efficiently on different types of problems. The ideal is to create a team system that allows professionals to belong to an interdisciplinary team and at the same time use other methods of practice with individuals, teams, or groups as needs dictate. Using the model (see Figure 2.5), a physician who belonged to an IHCT in a primary care clinic setting might meet briefly with a nurse and a physical therapist (ad hoc group) to discuss a hospitalized patient's needs for mobility while hospitalized. That same physician might attend a multidisciplinary planning conference (formal work group) in a nursing home once a week. The physician might meet monthly with a group of clinic staff physicians (unidisciplinary formal work group) to discuss policies relative to medical care. The physician might meet regularly with the other physicians who are on the interdisciplinary clinic team to discuss their ongoing relationship with each other and with the other health professionals on the team (unidisciplinary interactive team). The interdisciplinary clinic team will meet regularly to discuss patient care plans and will periodically meet to discuss the team's function.

Unfortunately, the meetings to discuss team function are often left in the dust as patient care pressures mount. Maintaining an IHCT system requires strong support from both administrators and clinicians. The costs of maintaining an IHCT can be easily estimated. However, those costs are usually compared to the direct costs of not maintaining an IHCT. It is much more difficult to estimate the longer term costs of not intervening in time to avert problems. It is also difficult to estimate the cost of a team that does not function well together. Despite the difficulties of doing so, costs for each of these situations must be factored into equations for efficiency of care. Given the issues discussed in this section, it is useful to consider how the care of Henry could have been delivered more efficiently.

The Case of Henry

A cardiologist prescribed three new medications for his new patient, Henry, a 70-year-old with unstable cardiac disease and hypertension. Henry told the cardiologist about his medications for diabetes but forgot to tell him about the other medications that were prescribed by his family doctor for depression and a seizure disorder. The clinic nurse gave Henry instructions for taking the three new medications. Henry procured the medicine at one pharmacy and the pharmacist gave him instructions on the medications and potential interactions between them. Henry ordered his other medications from another pharmacy that was not linked into the computer system of the first pharmacy. Some of those medications had potentially harmful interacting effects with Henry's initial medications but he was not instructed in those side effects.

Henry was involved with a community outreach social worker who discovered that he was not taking some of his medications because they interfered with his ability to leave his home at certain times of the day so he could visit the neighborhood restaurant to eat their famous "finger-lickin chicken" and "fudge-bottom pie." Additionally, Henry forgot to take his medicine before bed as he felt it was too difficult for him to make another trip down the stairs to get it. The social worker called a pharmacist to discuss all of the medications and to consult on a better way to fit the medication regimen into the patient's schedule. The social worker thought that consultations by an occupational therapist and a dietitian were necessary and called the clinic nurse who decided the patient needed to be seen again in the clinic. Before the patient could be scheduled he had an acute cardiac event and was hospitalized.

SUMMARY

Although the IHCT appears to be a simple and straightforward entity, in reality it is a complex phenomenon that requires intense efforts for development and maintenance. A well-functioning IHCT encompasses multiple methods of practice and achieves efficiency by applying a particular team method where and when it is needed (i.e., the least intense method required to accomplish the task). This chapter described a model of IHCT function and maintenance. It also outlined six methods of practice that, when understood and used, function as a system for providing efficient health care. The purpose of presenting this model is to urge you to strive for understanding rather than perfection. There is no expectation that members of an IHCT will remain in the performing phase. In fact, most of the time they will probably be elsewhere. However, it is only with an understanding of the components and phases of IHCT development that members of an IHCT can strive to achieve the team's ideal level of practice. When properly constructed and well functioning, the IHCT is a dynamic entity with ebbs and flows of development. An IHCT that attends to its development and that maintains a depth of culture is not only personally rewarding to team members, but it may also be the best hope to address the situational complexity of the current health care system.

Initially, this model may be difficult to understand. However, it is meant to be a learning tool that you can return to as questions arise in your team development experience. Although you may not master this model the first time you read it, use it to reflect on problems that develop in the teams with which you work. Eventually, it will help you understand the complexities of those problems and with that understanding you will be better able to devise solutions that will help your IHCT develop and strengthen its practice. The remaining chapters discuss in more detail some of the concepts introduced in this model.

NOTES

1. Drinka, T.J.K. (1991). A case study of leadership on a long term interdisciplinary health care team (Doctoral dissertation, University of Wisconsin-Madison, 1990). *Dissertation Abstracts International, 51:11*, 3599A.

2. Romig, D. A. (1996). *Breakthrough teamwork*. Chicago, IL: Irwin.

3. Drinka, T., & Ray, R. O. (1986). An investigation of power in an interdisciplinary health care team. *Gerontology & Geriatrics Education, 6*(3), 43–53.

4. Kaluzny, A. (1985). Design and management of disciplinary and interdisciplinary groups in health services: Review and critique. *Medical Care Review, 42*, 77–112.

5. Anderson, O., & Gevitz, N. (1983). The general hospital: A social and historical perspective. In D. Mechanic (Ed.), *Handbook of health, health care, and the health professions* (pp. 305– 317). New York: The Free Press.

6. Drinka, *A case study of leadership.*

7. Rittel, H., & Webber, M. (1973). Dilemmas in a general theory of planning. *Policy Sciences, 4*, 155–169.

3

Intangibles That Affect Team Development and Maintenance

Members of health care teams harbor images of the teams (past and present) on which they have served. Negative and positive experiences are remembered at both conscious and subconscious levels and undoubtedly affect how members do or do not engage with teammates. Images of teams are also a reflection of interpersonal experiences—past and present. These interpersonal experiences with family, friends, and acquaintances lay the groundwork for the way health care providers view themselves in relation to a team and for how quickly they assimilate into the team. The team experiences in which health providers engage as part of their training and work experience can be expressed in pictures, metaphors, and myths. In this chapter, we discuss how pictures, metaphors, and myths emerge, how they can affect members' views of the team, and how teams can use them to grow.

IHCTs in similar settings are not necessarily alike. When health care providers receive their training in one team setting and end up working in another they may be surprised to find that there are major team differences between the two settings. IHCTs take on their own unique characteristics and these perpetuate themselves over time. In this chapter, we review some of the different attributes of IHCTs in a variety of settings. We also address some of the differences and similarities that exist between IHCTs and self-directed work teams (SDWTs) in business settings.

HOW MEMBERS OF HEALTH CARE TEAMS VIEW TEAMS

Pictures

Viewed as a collective, the pictures that team members draw can present a valuable examination of their team. A team's collective pictures can indicate the extent of the team members' experience and understanding of teams in general and of their team in particular. In exercises conducted as part of team workshops in which we have been involved, team members were each asked to draw a picture of a health care team, not designating whether it was to be of the team on which they were currently serving or of a team on which they had previously served. Many of the pictures were noteworthy. Some were very detailed and some were simple drawings of one element of team function. Many of the pictures were poignant depictions of some team experience that was traumatic for the team member.

Occasionally, all members of a team have drawn pictures that gave glowing accounts of teamwork. Members of an IHCT that was in crisis drew pictures of flowers in bloom, people holding hands around a circle, smiling faces of team members and patients, and other positive images. Collectively, these pictures were not an accurate reflection of their team. They were not even a realistic impression of a well-functioning team. They raised an index of suspicion that the team members were unable to accurately view their team or were covering up normal conflicts that occur as part of teamwork. This "gloss of goodness" may also have been a reflection of the way their organization viewed the world. When each team member was asked to draw a picture of team conflict, some were unable to do so. Also, when prompted, most were able to picture at least one of the problems that regularly occurred on their team. Several members depicted the same conflict. This opened up the discussion and the team was able to progress in its development.

Having team members draw pictures of their team can also uncover problems within the team that are never discussed because of a lack of trust among team members. Many of the pictures that team members have drawn have been memorable. One team member who did not want to engage in team development activities (because she said that her team was doing just fine) drew a picture of the three monkeys that portray "hear no evil, see no evil, speak no evil" to represent her team. This picture indicated that the team member knew that the team was covering up problems and that it was the team's culture to do so.

The "three monkeys" is one of the pictures that team members have drawn often in workshops. It seems to portray an inability to face conflict.

Another common theme has been broken circles, indicating that there was no communication between team members, or a horse and a cart with no driver, indicating a lack of leadership. Pictures with team members crossing hurdles, jumping through fire, and climbing mountains have also been common. Another less common theme has been puzzles with pieces that fit together in different ways at different times, and sometimes not all of the pieces need to be used. When the pictures that team members draw are complex, having positive and negative elements in them, it is an indication that the team member has thought about the team's development and is trying to improve the team's work. The pictures that team members draw can be starting points for a team to evaluate its developmental process.

Metaphors

Metaphors are another mechanism for uncovering the views that health professionals have of their team or teams in general. Teams are everywhere. Health care professionals grew up, either as observers or participants, with varied team experiences: softball, volleyball, spelling, and debate teams. These team experiences plus life experiences in families and other more formal groups have etched metaphors of teams in our minds. Metaphors that health professionals collect during primary professional training may be altered once those individuals leave their training. Also, the metaphors continue to change by experiences that practitioners encounter in their work. Despite the fact that sports team metaphors are the metaphors to which we have most often been exposed, they do not appear to be the predominant team metaphors for health care professionals.

One study of metaphors that team members used to describe interdisciplinary health care teams found that health professionals who worked on teams generally applied more nonsports than sports metaphors to teamwork (e.g., music, learning, synergistic effects, and the weather). When team members did apply sports metaphors to teams, they often had differing interpretations of a particular sports metaphor. For example, the sports metaphor of football was seen by one team member as "teamwork with good coaches" and by another as "a bunch of unfriendly quarterbacks—too many directors—too few doers." Study respondents also reported using different metaphors in current practice than those they had used at the end of their formal professional training. One member noted that at the culmination of his training, his metaphor for team was "figure skating—all beauty, graceful and smooth with a few falls now and then, little did I know!" After several years of practice, this team member had changed his metaphor to, "a hockey team—there are fights within a team and between teams. There can be bruises (ego and physical) and disagreements, etc., but in the end it's team effort that wins." The diverse metaphors demonstrated that this individual, during his training, had a simplistic metaphor of team. However, his view of *team* matured with his practice experience as evidenced by his latter metaphor. Although this individual's later metaphor might be interpreted by some as negative, it reflected the complex nature of an IHCT.[1]

Observing the way team members use metaphors can be a valuable tool in diagnosing the state of a team. When team members apply unidimensional metaphors to dynamic and complex processes it is a clear sign that something is not working. Using unidimensional metaphors, like "a lovely flower in bloom," may indicate that either the team member is not integrated into the team or that the team is not well developed. When a unidimensional metaphor is negative, as "the patient is the puck," it may indicate that the team has unresolved conflict. Like the team member who changed from the figure skating to the hockey metaphor, the metaphors of team members should grow dimensionally as the team itself develops. Team members can be taught to be aware of the metaphors that they and other team members use and to use them as a measure of the team's developmental process. It is important for an IHCT to attain a common understanding of metaphors that are applied to the team by making them explicit and discussing their meanings. As a team process exercise, a team member might ask all team members to list their metaphors for the team. This could be done anonymously, openly, serially or collectively. It would be essential to discuss what the metaphors mean, whether or not a team likes their metaphors, and how the team would like to see them change over time.

Myths

Myths and legends are stories that arise in the course of a team's development. Myths unmask the "worldview" of the team's members or of the team as a whole. Myths and legends are a powerful force that teams can use to develop and sustain a particular culture. One of the reasons myths are so powerful is that they tap into stories that were presented to us as children. One myth involves a powerful figure that has the capacity to save people from distress. One IHCT had been struggling for a year to develop its clinical base. In the course of that development it had a formal leader who did not establish a firm direction for the team. The team was just beginning to develop its informal leadership roles. Suddenly, a powerful physician was hired to be the team's director at a time when the team's funding was in jeopardy. This physician was able to reestablish the funding and evolved as the team's protector. The team members referred to him as "big daddy" and whenever members needed something they would go to him knowing that they would be listened to.

An IHCT was assigned a director who was a powerful physician in the larger organization and was feared by many members of the team. One day, two team members were walking down the hospital corridor and passed the team director who was speaking to a group of students. He bellowed down the hall at them, "Don't you stop and say hello to god?" Although it was the director's way of making a joke, it was clear that he saw himself as powerful. Because many team members did not feel free to approach this director they often let team business slide. Team conflicts that should have been addressed were ignored and the team began to collapse.

Perhaps a team has struggled collectively against a system that had little faith in the team's ability to manage a particular type of patient. If the health care team proves successful at providing good care to those patients who were deemed unsalvageable by the system, a myth might develop about that team. That team might also see itself as able to perform superhuman feats. One health care team saw itself as a low flying plane, able to evade the radar of bureaucratic rules that the organization imposed to keep change from occurring. Within the system the team was seen as a maverick, not accepted by most but secretly admired and envied.

One IHCT harbored a myth of limitless creativity. The team was sure that it could solve any complex problem that came its way. It was caring for a particularly difficult 90-year-old patient. This person had diabetes, dementia, congestive heart failure, and multiple other problems. He was demanding constant attention from his family caregivers and was wearing them out. The team was expending inordinate amounts of energy and resources to find ways to keep the patient and family satisfied. The patient's son became very frustrated at the effect his father's constant care had on his mother. At a particularly frustrating time he asked a team member if they couldn't just give his father a pill to make him better. Rather than realizing their limits, the team began struggling even harder to find a solution to this situation. During a team meeting, members were re-examining the patient's medications and questioning once again their approach when one of the team members threw a foot-long plastic pill on the table. The team burst out laughing as they realized that they were beyond realistic limits of patient care. For the moment, the myth of invincibility was exploded but it would take ongoing work to break through the team's fantasy that they were magicians.

The important thing to note about pictures, metaphors, and myths is that they are often implicit and remain unquestioned. Over time, they become reified and part of a team's culture. Sometimes these images are positive and help the team develop and meet its goals. However, these images can also be destructive to the team's development and may impede team growth. Taking time to make a team's images explicit is a good team development exercise and can help a team see why it is headed in the direction of its mission or, conversely, why it might have strayed off course.

DIFFERING CULTURES OF HEALTH CARE TEAMS: PRIMARY CARE, REHABILITATION, GERIATRICS, MENTAL HEALTH, AND HOME CARE

Discussing cultures of any kind can be dangerous as one may be accused of stereotyping. However, in our experience, there appears to be a difference in the way different types of IHCTs develop and in the values that they hold about how to behave. Just as populations in different parts of a city or in different areas of a country develop unique ways of behaving, in health care different cultures emerge in various subspecialty departments. Also, different types of IHCTs in health care settings may attract certain personality types and people who share unique goals and values for delivering care.

Primary Care

IHCTs in primary care tend to attract individuals who want to focus on the human touch. Rather than rigorous detail, they are primarily attracted to variety in the types of patients they see and problems they address. The difficulty is in knowing what to treat, how much to treat, and when to refer. Primary care IHCTs tend to have fewer core disciplines, usually physicians and nurses with a mental health worker like a social worker or psychologist. Having a greater variety of disciplines available would enable the primary care IHCT to make decisions with greater accuracy. However, because this is not seen as economically feasible, the primary care IHCT must learn to bring other disciplines into their team as consultants or temporary members. It is vital for them to learn skills in interteam communication. In some primary care settings there is a trend toward hiring lesser skilled workers (e.g., nursing assistants or licensed practical nurses), to perform more of the work. However, if the team does not establish procedures and training for communication between different levels of providers, members have difficulty knowing their limits and when and how to use the skills of the other team members. In this case, the team is unable to reap the economic benefits of having multiple levels of providers.

Rehabilitation

IHCTs in rehabilitation departments focus on intense treatment and rapid turnover. Although the team may have multiple levels of providers, team members are usually well trained in their disciplines. In acute and subacute settings the physician is commonly the unquestioned leader of the team. These teams tend to focus on team structure and not on team process issues because team process is not a focus of physician training. Individuals are trained to do specific tasks although different professions may informally share some tasks. Each discipline reports their findings to the team and the physician makes the decisions. Rehabilitation teams in general could benefit from training in team process, especially the use of informal leadership and constructive confrontation to increase efficiency and worker satisfaction.

Geriatrics

IHCTs in geriatric settings tend to evaluate and treat frail patients with complex and interacting physical and psychosocial problems. Because of these patient characteristics, team members should be highly trained professionals. Unfortunately, this is not always the case. In fact, IHCTs in geriatric settings may be just the opposite because administrators have a habit of assigning staff, who were problems in other departments, to the most chronic care team "where they can do the least harm."

In long-term care settings, team members may be unskilled workers or lesser skilled professionals. This presents a problem because in a setting where team members other than the physician should take over leadership roles, team members may not have the skills to do so and either weak or autocratic leadership may emerge. Geriatrics IHCTs, like the two previously mentioned types of teams, do not necessarily like to take the time to work on team process issues. However, when skilled professionals are assigned to work in geriatric IHCTs they have the capacity to create teams of greatness. Health care providers who receive team training in geriatrics do not assume that the physician must be "the leader" of the team. They learn to develop many leaders with different leadership skills and to promote different types of leadership where and when it is needed.

Mental Health

IHCTs in mental health settings are comprised of psychiatrists, social workers, psychologists, nurses, activity therapists, and counselors. They focus on the emotional aspects of patients, relying on consults from other physicians and allied health professionals for problems that are not of a mental health nature. Of all team types, mental health team members are the best trained to address the process issues of teams. This is both an asset and a liability. They have the capacity to assure that the team achieves a high level of functioning. However, because they are so skilled at understanding psychological interactions, they are also skilled at using them to avoid conflict situations that could propel the team to greater heights of function. They value decision making by consensus and will take time to assure that every member is heard. In assuring that everyone on the team has an equal say, they may get bogged down in values and ethical dilemmas, extending the time for resolving clinical issues. In general, mental health IHCTs need to work on increasing their efficiency in decision making without compromising their ability to confront conflict.

Home Care and Treatment

Home care teams are diverse and new models are continually emerging. Generally home care teams are comprised of several levels of nursing staff (e.g., registered nurses, licensed practical nurses, nursing assistants, and nurse practitioners). Home care teams also have physical and occupational therapists, social workers, speech pathologists, chore workers, and personal care workers. The physician may function as a consultant and may attend few patient care meetings. Because their work is physically diffused in the community, the providers on this type of team are frequently autonomous thinkers who are not inclined to see the need to collaborate. Although this trait is helpful in many situations these team members encounter, it is an impediment when they are working with very complex patient conditions. Home care teams have a critical need to develop systems for integrative problem setting and for ongoing communication. And although these teams can benefit from the technology of computers and portable phones, they are teams that need to be highly developed and whose members need to be trained in the process skills of communication. When there are conflicts between members on home care teams, it is all too easy to ignore them until they become major problems. An additional problem in home care teams is the need to develop trust between different levels of providers with whom members may have little in-person contact.

Despite the varied cultures that exist in IHCTs from different settings, all IHCTs have one thing in common (i.e., a need for team development and maintenance activities). It is critical for all IHCTs to focus on their strengths and to address their weaknesses on an ongoing basis. The organization must allow them time for periodic review of their team function. The organization can also help assure that teams are evaluating their function in line with the team and the organization's goals for care.

DIFFERENCES AND SIMILARITIES BETWEEN INTERDISCIPLINARY HEALTH CARE TEAMS AND SDWTs IN BUSINESS

It is important to look at SDWTs in business settings because they have a history that is comparable to IHCTs. Also, most of the administrators of health care organizations have been trained in a business culture and have brought that culture into health care. Successful SDWTs have interdependent members, a shared goal or mission, climate of trust, open and honest communication, sense of belonging, consensus decision making, and participative leadership. Diversity is valued as an asset and creativity and risk-taking are encouraged. An SDWT develops the ability to self-correct by examining its processes and practices.[2]

Differences

IHCTs differ from SDWTs in business by virtue of their members, definition of consumer, and nature of their "product." Many of the theories developed for work teams in nonhealth care settings present problems when applied to IHCTs (e.g., the presence of physicians on IHCTs, the patient's relationship to the health care team, and the uncertain nature of physical and mental health).

Presence of physicians and other autonomous disciplines. IHCTs are unique among work teams because health care requires involvement by physicians. In the United States, by tradition, physicians have the highest level of training; the most ascribed power; and in the medical literature they are unquestioningly referred to as the team leader.[3] The relative high status of physicians coupled with the learned expectations of other health professionals establishes a double bind. This expectation of physician leadership plays out in several ways. Despite the fact that some physicians may incorporate this expectation of their leadership, they may have limited time and heavy commitments that prevent them from executing their presumed leadership roles. The team's members may also expect that a physician will assume a formal leadership role when the physician has no intention of doing so. The patient complicates this game of chance because the nature of a patient's problems might require assumption of a leadership role by team members who are not physicians. IHCTs and SDWTs have members from autonomous disciplines with specialized education and unique languages. Separatist attitudes that exist among professionals from different disciplines, especially in times of stress, may promote rejection of leaders from other disciplines and impede openness, innovation, and constructive confrontation in addressing complex problems. However, health care is unique in the implied status of physicians and the uncertainty of their relationship to the IHCT.

Patient's relationship to the IHCT. The role that patients want to play in their health care is as complex as the health care itself. It involves emotion, willingness to teach and learn, and assurances of understanding. Like team members who simplify team concepts, patients try to simplify their health care so they can understand it. Although patients are not necessarily part of an ongoing team, they are central to the team's role. Patients may have to be invited to participate in their care and for the length of their care will be involved with some of the team's activities. Patients may not want to listen to the complex interactions that are potentiated by multiple therapies that may be required for their care. Understanding the sometimes conflicting interplay of patient emotion and intellect is at the heart of the IHCT's work. The most difficult interactions often come at a time when a patient is least likely to understand and is the most vulnerable to being misunderstood by the team.

Patients are not customers in a business sense, and this presents ethical issues for the IHCT. Patients may be well informed and know what they want. However, patients may also be very well informed and not have the emotional stability to make a reasonable decision. Sometimes patients may be presented with an array of unpalatable options. They cannot decide what they want, nor do they know what is best for them. Also, illness may block even an assertive person's ability to get the information necessary to make good health care decisions.

Uncertain nature of physical and mental health. The uncertainty of the outcome often adds weight to the ethical dilemmas that face the team. In general, health is an extremely complex entity. Physical symptoms are mediated by psychological state and vice versa. Many conditions are interacting and have no easy cures. Additionally, what is viewed as a cure by one person may not be by another. Advances in health care remedies and technology seem to come almost daily. And for every change there is a potential interaction with an existing remedy or technology. There are few places in business where daily decisions in an uncertain environment have direct impact on the life or death of another person. Health care professionals take this responsibility very seriously. This need to "not make a mistake" in an uncertain area places pressures on members of IHCTs that are different from those placed on members of most SDWTs.

There are additional differences between IHCTs and SDWTs. SDWTs in business settings appear to focus more on teaching skills that promote interaction with the broader organization.[4] Because of their interests in "continuous improvement," SDWTs also promote learning a technical base for evaluation. Additionally, SDWTs often promote cross training and the learning of self-management techniques by all team members. On the other hand, IHCTs have better addressed issues related to interprofessional differences. They do not attempt to cross-train health providers from different disciplines. However, they do help members recognize and capitalize on areas of skill overlap. Rather than focus on time-consuming management skills, IHCTs address functional leadership and help members assume appropriate leadership roles.[5]

Similarities

Despite the differences between IHCTs and SDWTs there are also many similarities. During the 1980s and 1990s, a newer sector of health care was developing its own concept of teams. Health care managers increasingly emerged from the business community and schools of health care management. These individuals had been trained in the business model of teamwork. Although they were taught to believe in teams, they held different images of "team" from those held by health professionals. As their worlds merge with those of health professionals, health care and business teams are becoming more alike.

Continual existence of entering and leaving members. The continual existence of entering and leaving members is a problem for both IHCTs and SDWTs in business. IHCTs seldom choose their members, and it is common for members to terminate and new members to join. The structure of health care systems encourages high staff turnover and rotating key disciplines like nursing. Health care administrators may borrow staff from one specialized team to cover shortages in another specialized team. SDWTs cover these inevitabilities by cross training. In health care, coverage is just expected. Like SDWTs in business settings, IHCTs are subject to downsizing. Frequent transfers in organizational priorities often result in changes in external funding for health care and a hesitancy to pay for primary patient support services by disciplines such as social work, dietetics, or occupational therapy. Urgent patient care tasks and the lack of time for team development activities in health settings prohibit the entire IHCT from meeting the needs of each new member. And finally, although SDWTs talk about team development, like IHCTs they usually do not take the time to meet the needs of new members.

Bi-level or incongruous development. As a result of changing personal, professional, and team issues—including moderate to high membership turnover—an IHCT and a SDWT have at least two developmental levels: (a) the level of the team and (b) the level of the individual member.

Lacoursiere[6] concluded that in a group, isolated individuals can reflect phases differing from the group's developmental phase. Based on our discussions with members of a variety of IHCTs and SDWTs, it appears common for individual members to reflect different phases of development from the team as a whole. It is expected that new IHCT members will be at different developmental phases from the rest of the IHCT. Also, ongoing members may regress to earlier phases or simply not move as rapidly through the phases as other members.

SUMMARY

Although it might seem odd for health care professionals to dwell on their mental images, myths, and metaphors, taking time to explore them can enhance their ability to communicate with other team members and in turn can improve their team practice. Health care providers learn quickly to work hard, to produce, and to avoid mistakes. It is difficult to break through this veneer of hard work and caring in order to explore a problem that the team is having. The use of mental images, myths, and metaphors is a powerful mechanism that can help an IHCT overcome its barriers to learning and efficiency of practice. Understanding how IHCTs might differ from other organizational team cultures can also be useful in interacting with those cultures to enhance the work of the IHCT. As the culture of a business model envelops health care, it is important for IHCTs to realize why they are different and what members can use from both worlds to improve patient care and the well-being of colleagues.

NOTES

1. Drinka, T.J.K., & Miller, T. F. (1996). The health care team as metaphor: A preliminary study. *Journal of Allied Health*, *25*(3), 247–261.

2. Orsburn, J. D., Moran, L., Musselwhite, E., & Zenger, J. H. (1990). *Self-directed work teams: The new American challenge*. Homewood, IL: Business One Irwin.

3. Charatan, F. B., Foley, C. J., & Libow, L. S. (1985). The team approach to geriatric medicine. In R. Andres, E. L. Bierman, & W. R. Hazzard (Eds.), *Principles of geriatric medicine* (pp. 169–175). New York: McGraw-Hill.

4. Drinka, T.J.K. (1996). Applying learning from self-directed work teams in business to curriculum development for interdisciplinary geriatric teams. *Educational Gerontology*, *22*, 433–450.

5. Drinka, T.J.K. (1991). Development and maintenance of an interdisciplinary health care team: A case study. *Gerontology & Geriatrics Education*, *12*(1), 111–127.

6. Lacoursiere, R. B. (1980). *The life cycle of groups: Group development stage theory*. New York: Human Sciences Press.

4

Communicating in Teamwork: Understanding Professional Differences and Their Implications for Working Together

Effective teamwork requires good communication. Frustrated team members often express concerns about its quality and extent. As in any relationship between people, the ability to "keep the lines of communication open" in an IHCT is an important indicator of effective teamwork skills. In IHCTs, the dimensions of communication most often discussed relate to issues involving personality clashes, role overlap and conflict, and the effective use and sharing of clinically important information. Absent is an examination of underlying problems with communication based on the professional differences among health care providers, including how they acquired particular values over the course of their education and subsequent clinical work experience. These values are related to their orientations both to the patient and toward each other.

For example, physicians tend to approach patients within a predominantly biomedical model, emphasizing "objective" information from laboratory tests as a means to focus on increasingly narrow interpretations of the patient's "problem." Most nurses, however, tend to have a much broader view of the "patient as person," which includes his or her interpretation of the meaning of the illness and its significance for everyday living. This more holistic approach to the patient's problem embodies more qualitative dimensions, in contrast with the medical emphasis on quantitative, "factual" data as sufficient to understanding the problem. Unless these values and the assumptions of their relative importance are made clear, physicians and nurses may have difficulty working together on an IHCT—because each has different views of professional priorities and the basic values that create these priorities.

Also, with the present sweeping changes in the health care system, it is increasingly important for health care professionals to understand how their own roles are shifting in response to forces emphasizing cost containment and quality improvement. Although most health care providers have been trained to believe that their particular role and disciplinary focus are unique, in fact there is substantial overlap in certain areas among many health professions. For example, both nursing and social work focus on psychosocial dimensions of patient care, although the extent and depth of this emphasis vary. Greater willingness to be flexible, collaborative, and cooperative is the hallmark of the new health care system that is emerging from current forces at work—a willingness assuming increased ability to communicate about roles, values, and styles of practice.

These issues involving communication are the focus of this chapter. In particular, we examine how the powerful influence of professional socialization—the process of acquiring an identity as a physician, nurse, or social worker—can affect the overall outlook and personal sense of self of the health care provider. Especially important are the particular values and overall value orientations instilled in this process—including those related to such ethical concepts as autonomy and quality of life—that play a crucial role in establishing and shaping these emerging professional identities. Subsequent to initial education, the experiences of clinicians in the workplace and their exposure to different types of patients, problems, and other professionals can further mold their sense of self as a professional. Indeed, as the effects of a changing health care system continue to be felt in the workplace and in the professional identities of providers, there will be increasing impact of the practice setting on changes in how health care providers see themselves and others in relation to the IHCT.

The main message in this chapter is a call for the adoption of a "reflective ethic" of interdisciplinary teamwork practice; that is, health care providers working in collaborative settings need to become more aware of how their own professional backgrounds, training, and work experience and relationships have shaped who they are and how they think. They must also become more aware of the differences between themselves and their fellow team members from different backgrounds. All too often, however, the reality of clinical practice—with its demands for making important assessment and care plan decisions about patients under severe time and resource constraints—makes the luxury of developing such a perspective beyond the reach of many.

However, just as team members need time free from clinical pressures to reflect on "how they are doing" as a team, so too do they need the time to develop the reflective skills necessary for acquiring an appreciation of each other, their unique backgrounds and training, and individual perspectives on clinical decision making that make professions distinctive. In this sense, the "reflective team" is the analogue of the "learning team," which is open to sharing information and perspectives, addressing group concerns and issues, and educating its members and the patient about important issues to be considered in any clinical decision-making process.

In this chapter, we discuss these issues, first, by developing an understanding of what is meant by the term *professional socialization* and how we become who we are in the process of being educated and gaining work experience in a particular health care profession. Second, the implications of this training for the type of identity and outlook within which a health care professional operates are considered. In the previous example, the extent to which a profession adopts a more limited, "biomedical" model versus a more holistic approach to the patient as a person is centrally important in this discussion. Third and finally, we examine the specific clinical implications of these differences among professionals. In particular, how clinical problems are defined and addressed, how quality of life is conceptualized, and how patterns of communication among health care professionals are affected in collaborative settings are discussed.

Overall, the issues involving communication on IHCTs are complicated, but we hope that this chapter helps sort them out, develops a framework for thinking about them, and provides some new insights into previously unaddressed dimensions of this important topic. The ability to reflect on the important differences, as well as the similarities, among the health professions—as well as to understand how these factors are changing in the face of forces transforming our health care system—is an increasingly important characteristic of effective teamwork and collaboration for the future of the health professions.

BECOMING A HEALTH CARE PROFESSIONAL: HOW EDUCATION AND SOCIALIZATION SHAPE WHO WE ARE

Becoming a health care provider means acquiring the knowledge, skills, values, roles, and attitudes associated with the practice of a particular profession. The very fact that there are different health care professions suggests that each health care discipline tends to see itself as unique in the nature of the basic practice framework into which its students are inducted, trained, and credentialed—as well as in the workplace and clinical practice settings in which they subsequently work. This process is in many respects similar to how different cultures socialize their members into the unique ways of thinking and acting that characterize them, based on shared views of the world, guidelines for individual action, and collective values that bind the community together.

Extending this metaphor to health professions education offers fresh insight into how new "inductees" in health professions training programs are usually protectively housed in different buildings on campus—called colleges or schools—where they can be free from the potentially contaminating and threatening influences of students and faculty from other fields. Similar courses may be taught independently for students in different health sciences programs, reinforcing the relative insularity and parochialism of educational processes at the university or college level. The acquisition of unique patterns of language, modes of dress and demeanor, and norms of behavior are all outward manifestations of this inward transformation. Indeed, some commentators have even argued that exposure of students to health disciplines different from their own would only serve to confuse them and threaten their emerging sense of identity. Only when the student is sufficiently socialized into this identity do we allow him or her to have clinical contact with other professions, usually following graduation.

Professional Isolation in Higher Education

Ever notice how faculty and students from different departments or disciplines tend to sit together at meetings and courses?

In our interdisciplinary team health promotion course, we noted at the beginning of the semester that students from nursing, pharmacy, and nutrition would sit together in their own groups based on profession. However, as the semester proceeded, these tight groups began to break down, with more intermingling and seating based on other factors, such as wanting to talk to each other, personality characteristics, and so on. As faculty we knew we were making progress when students started breaking out of their comfortable, disciplinary groupings!

Moreover, in their personal journals—required as a part of the course—the participants wrote about their limited experience in working with students from other health professions. For example, many nursing students had never worked before with a pharmacy or dietetics student. They soon began to realize that these students were in many ways "just like them," but that they had important additional information to contribute to improving patient care.

Even in the case of new paraprofessional disciplines, such as nurses aides, there is a tendency for the more limited technical training orienting these workers to their role in the health care system to reinforce some of the same role divisions observed in the more extensively educated professions. Moreover, the effects of the workplace on the identity formation of such paraprofessionals tend to channel them into "acceptable" patterns of behavior and assumptions of relative status.

SOCIALIZATION AS IDENTITY AND VALUE FORMATION

Socialization may be conceptualized as a developmental process, much like the way in which we think of individual human development along the life course. In this sense, it may be characterized as a continual interaction between the individual and his or her environment, by accord and discord between what is expected and what is actually experienced, and by the active creation of meaning by the individual. Seen from this perspective, socialization may be compared with theories of cognitive and moral development, in which the individual develops linkages between the "ways of knowing" information and acquiring knowledge, and the "principles of behaving" that guide individual behavior. Socialization thus becomes a more active process of "self-concept or identity creation" than the more passive one of learning appropriate social roles.

The process of socialization extends well beyond the period of formal education and training. Although its powerful influence may begin while the student is in a formal career-preparation period, such as a degree program, socialization continues on into the workplace. The powerful effects of organizational contexts, fellow workers and colleagues, supervisors, and experiences with patients and their families in the clinical setting further define professional roles, identities, values, and orientations. As already mentioned, forces creating changes in the organization of health care systems can cause shifts in professional roles, identities, and patterns of practice. For example, managed care has increased the focus on primary care and decreased the emphasis on specialty clinics. These changes have had effects on professional roles and responsibilities. For example, the profession of nursing has assumed more of the roles associated with other disciplines (such as social work) as a direct result of these developments within the health care system.

Socialization may also be seen as the development of a unique voice, perspective, or personal and professional view of the world. The metaphor of "voice" has been applied to differing health care providers working in collaborative settings.[1] Carol Gilligan[2] argued, for example, that women possess a unique moral voice of caring and connection, in contrast with the more rule-based approach typical of men. In solving moral dilemmas, women may emphasize more the importance of maintaining connectedness than the simple application of ethical principles. Similarly, patients and providers have different voices because of the different worlds of the individual and the professional they inhabit.[3]

Identity Formation on Interdisciplinary Teams

In our years of offering interdisciplinary health professions courses, we have found that students often come into the experience with "pat" explanations and simplistic conceptions of their professional identities.

However, when they are placed in settings where some role overlap exists—such as between nursing and dietetics students with regard to patient nutrition education—the are forced to confront the questions about who they really are and what they really do. Initially defensive in situations where they think they each have a unique role, the students eventually come to recognize that there is overlap in the health professions and that this is alright. Ultimately, they come away with a stronger sense of who they are and the roles they play in the health care system.

Values may be considered as one of the essential "building blocks" of this identity formation process. Here, values represent meanings and the basis for internalized norms and standards of the professional culture characteristic of the individual's own behavior and self-concept. Values become the basis for the life themes or stories we tell to make sense of our lives. "Through life stories, people 'account' for their lives, that is, they make them logical and coherent and imbue them with a sense of naturalness and rightness. They select, define, classify, and organize experience in order to express the reality of their lives and permeate that reality with meaning."[4] Values based on early, formative stages in the lives of health care professionals may be carried with them into their selection of certain fields, thus continuing a "life story" into the professional domain. For example, research on physicians indicates that certain psychodynamic factors seem to underlie the choice of students to go into the field of medicine.[5] Early experiences with disease, conflicts, and troubled childhoods seem to be characteristic of physicians.

SOCIALIZATION AS AN INTERACTIVE AND VALUE-BASED PROCESS

The twin hallmarks of socialization are interaction and reflection. Professional identity is formed by the reciprocal interaction between the self and the environment, whether individual or institutional. As a student, the trainee's emergent identity is influenced by interactions with faculty, other students, and patients. As the student moves beyond formal education into the workplace, socialization continues with changing work environments;

new supervisors, colleagues, and patients; and the inevitable unexpected challenges, problems, and dilemmas that confront any health care professional.

To a large extent, the shaping effects of these new experiences and environments will depend on the degree of self-reflection attained by the individual. As Schön[6] suggested, professional practice consists of both the scientific aspects—those dependent on the technical knowledge and skills of a discipline—and the artistic aspects—those related to the ability to grapple with the gray areas of professional practice where moral ambiguity, value conflicts, and ethical dilemmas are commonplace. The reflective practitioner is able to recognize and tolerate the uncertainties, ambiguities, and limitations of actual practice—in short, to recognize that all knowledge and skill are limited and defined by the boundaries imposed by values. The reflective practitioner cannot be on "automatic pilot" in daily practice, numbed by the routines of clinical care and unconscious to the nuances based on value conflicts that characterize everyday life in current health care practice.

The Reflective Practitioner in Geriatrics

In the field of geriatrics, recent research by Kaufman[7] highlighted the importance of recognizing and naming the dilemmas implicit in practice as value conflicts in which the right course of action is not readily apparent—whether dealing with concerns about risk, autonomy, or advocacy. For example, how does the health care provider respond to a mentally competent elderly patient who wants to place him or herself at substantial risk by remaining at home in an unsafe environment, despite reservations on the part of the provider and the family? This is the classic ethical conflict between safety and autonomy that is so characteristic of clinical practice with older adults.

Extending the metaphor of the reflective practitioner, one can argue that truly reflective health care providers are aware not only of how their own training and socialization have affected the development of their clinical practice values—but also of how the education of others creates in them differing, yet perhaps complementary, value systems. Differences among medicine, nursing, and social work, for example, can be traced to influences unique to the professional training and socialization patterns of each discipline, as the next section explores in more detail.

BECOMING A PHYSICIAN, NURSE, OR SOCIAL WORKER: HOW AND WHY ARE THESE PROFESSIONS DIFFERENT?

As already discussed, the very existence of distinct health care professions is related to the fact that there are different bodies of knowledge to be learned, types of technical skills to be mastered, and value orientations to be acquired in the course of becoming a physician, nurse, or social worker. These three disciplines have been chosen for discussion primarily because of the well-developed literature describing their professional bases, patterns of socialization, and practice differences; however, the same principles apply equally well to other health care professions. In each case, much is known about the effects that this training has on the kind of health care professional each student is in the process of becoming. Although we must avoid stereotyping each profession, there are indeed striking patterns that do seem to characterize the ways in which different disciplines approach the patient, as well as each other—and these differences are important in clinical practice. However, there is also growing recognition that there may be substantial overlap in some of the core bodies of knowledge that underlie different health professions; for example, both social workers and nurses master similar knowledge on the psychosocial dimensions of practice, though the extent and depth of actual clinical skills in this area may differ.

Medicine: Forces of Depersonalization, Decontextualization, and Dehumanization

Medical education and socialization can be characterized as locked in an uneven power struggle between two very different value systems: one more reductionistic and scientific, the other more social and humanistic.[8] The former entails faith in the rational solution of medical problems, disinterested concern for the patient and society, and dedication to competency in practice and the standards of science. Because of these values, this perspective discounts the social, behavioral, and personal dimensions of illness; relegates familial and social dimensions of practice to the periphery; and dismisses ethical issues as simply "matters of opinion" not easily resolved by rational discourse.

In contrast, the more humanistic perspective on the practice of medicine considers the social and behavioral approaches to be as relevant as the biological; selects students for training on the basis of their social concerns and interests in people; emphasizes caring as much as curing; and considers the community—and not just the hospital—as the proper place for medical education. This aspect is obviously more holistic in its approach to the patient as a person; and, in the distinction made by Schön, is more apt to emphasize the value dimensions of practice than its more scientific aspects.

Scientific basis. Although there have been periodic calls for greater emphasis on the latter model of medical education, recent history suggests the overwhelming ascendancy of the former. Scientific methods have had growing centrality in medical care—for example, the use of large amounts of objective laboratory data—with a resultant erosion in direct patient contact.[9] Emphasizing the scientific basis for medicine enhances its professional legitimacy, but this outcome comes at the high cost of widening the distance separating the physician from the patient. Furthermore, the development of elaborate classification systems for diseases and illnesses downplays the variability among patients, objectifies medical practice, and reduces the real need to know patients and understand the unique meanings they ascribe to their conditions.

Medical socialization and moral development. Biases affecting the selection of students for medical training provide a good foundation for acquiring the characteristics inculcated in students once they actually get to medical school. Some research, for example, suggests that medical students are preselected for certain traits (such as narcissism) that negatively affect their abilities to be empathic and sensitive to the needs and concerns of others.[10] Moreover, other research has found that as students progress through medical school, they tend to develop preferences for healthy over sick patients.[11] Research already mentioned draws attention to the underlying psychodynamic forces that seem to characterize students who choose medicine over other professions.[12]

Additionally, studies of moral development in medical students reveal that their training inhibits the development of ethical reasoning.[13] Other observers suggest that although medical students may be drawn to the profession originally because of their care and concern for the patient, their "moral landscape" is reformed as a result of the training process.[14] This may be due in part to the need to develop detached concern as a protection from intense emotional responses to pain and suffering, as well as to the cognitive burden of processing vast amounts of scientific material.

Physician attitudes toward patients. Perhaps the most important desensitizing and dehumanizing period in medical education is the time of internship and residency training. This period may be characterized as one of "reality shock," where there is a transition between medical school—where there is more idealism in caring for the whole patient—and internship and residency—where time limitations and practice demands set severe restrictions on clinical practice.[15] Indeed, there is the development of "GROPing" ("getting rid of patients") behavior by residents and interns, in which physical and psychological distancing techniques are mastered to separate the physicians-in-training from patients and their families.[16] GROPing techniques include passing patients "down the hierarchy" to the least experienced, most junior members of the clinical team for patient care or education responsibilities; transfering patients laterally to social workers, whose formal role is associated with getting rid of patients; and narrowing the focus of interaction with the patient, such as a sharply focused history-taking session with emphasis on efficient data collection.

Going to the Doctor

Many older people report that when they go to the doctor, the doctor seems rushed and unable to really sit down and talk to the patients about their problems and questions. Moreover, these patients feel that when the doctor does talk to them, a lot of big words—jargon—are used that they don't understand. The focus in the discussion often seems to be on the "problems" and not the "person"—on the narrow medical issues but not on the big picture of the person's overall life and what it means to them.

I have seen this in action myself when I take my elderly mother to her doctor. He is concerned with her weight, blood pressure, osteoporosis, medications, and so on; but he never asks generally how she feels, how often she gets out with friends, or what her mental outlook is. So, I always try to inject some information about her daily lifestyle, activity levels, and state of mind. It is not that he is disinterested—it is just that he doesn't think of these things initially as the most important issues. Moreover, I find myself "translating" his medical "language" into "kitchen English" that is more readily understandable by my mother.

It is in these kinds of encounters that the medical view of the world becomes most apparent, and most problematic for older persons (and, indeed, all patients!).

The significance of this history-taking method has been studied, and it has been noted that the nature of the language and discourse—or "talk"—between doctor and patient is the main ingredient in medical care and the very foundation on which treatment and care goals are built.[17] Language analysis applied to the medical interview reveals that there is a wide cultural gap between the life world of the patient and the scientific-technological domain of the physician.[18] The two distinct voices of medicine and the patient represent different "provinces of meaning" or "modes of consciousness" that limit the physician's ability to understand and appreciate the patient's real-world concerns and life goals.

Nursing: Values of Patient as Person

Some of the same issues previously mentioned in the medical socialization literature are also present in nursing, such as reality shock between initial education and exposure to the real world of actual clinical practice. Additionally, the issue of values and value conflicts is frequently mentioned in the nursing socialization literature. Overall, the growing ability to deal with value conflicts is seen as an integral part of the nursing socialization process and, indeed, as central to the ability of nurses to become empathic and sensitive to the dilemmas at the core of nursing practice. Some observers, for example, clearly distinguish between the acquisition of critical thinking and problem-solving skills, and the internalization of certain values essential to the development of a professional nursing identity.

Values acquisition and transformation in nursing. The relation between the development of nursing identity and the acquisition of specific values has been studied, and it has been noted that human dignity is the core value constituting nurses' identity and guiding their practice with patients.[19] Other patient-related values—such as security, integrity, personhood, being a fellow human, autonomy, privacy, reciprocal trust, hope, and general humanity—all either arise from it or are aimed at its preservation.

A complementary approach to understanding how values are transformed during the nursing socialization process is based on the changing perceptions by nursing students of those for whom they are caring.[20] Coming to understand patients as people—people who are being cared about and not simply cared for—is viewed as an integral part of the maturity of the students as both nurses and adults. This shift in thinking is dependent on a set of transformational experiences growing out of nursing training, in which students increasingly identify with their patients as people. The process of reflection is a key element in this transformation in the understanding of "what it means to be a nurse."

Holistic approaches and models. Overall, it seems apparent that the education of nurses leads them to develop a more holistic approach to the patient—one less reductionistic and more humanistic than the medical model discussed previously. Indeed, within nursing itself new models are emerging to support this more holistic approach, linked to an understanding of the unique value priorities, meanings, hopes, and dreams of the patient.

Parse,[21] for example, put forward a model of nursing emphasizing the essential unity of the individual, in which the focus is on the lived experience and personal history of the patient—embodying personal values, concerns, and life goals. An integral part of nursing practice is the incorporation of an ethic of caring that places the patient at the very center of what nursing is all about: the lived world, the life story, and the goals of the patient become the essence of caring for and about the patient. This approach is in contrast with the old, problem-centered methodologies of assessment and care plan development controlled by the professional, in which the origin and perspective of nursing lie with the nurse.

Although one may distinguish these trends in nursing in general, one must still keep in mind that nursing as a profession is not monolithic. Differing educational specializations within nursing create relative emphases that are different; for example, nurse practitioners are more aligned with the biomedical model of health care, whereas clinical nurse specialists have a broader base and a more holistic approach to the patient. Different philosophies and approaches have led to conflicts within the nursing profession itself over appropriate models of care.

Social Work: Socialization for Advocacy and Empowerment

The socialization of social workers is sometimes contrasted with that of physicians. For example, social workers are taught the importance of dealing with feelings and relationships, and mentors in the social work education process emphasize the development of self-awareness and conscious use of the self in transactions with others.[22] Similarly, the more stable, long-term contact and interrelationships between social work students and their supervisors—as well as between social workers and their patients—are in stark contrast with the rapid rotational changes that sever growing bonds of connection for medical students. Additionally, social workers are taught to broaden the basis for clinical decision making, to "rule in" dimensions of problems that may be initially overlooked in assessments—such as the psychosocial and economic dimensions of illness—rather than the more traditional "ruling out" of information in the medical diagnostic process.[23]

"Ruling In" and "Ruling Out" Problems

A classic example of how physicians and social workers differ is illustrated in a fairly typical case discussion about an older woman who was not taking her medications properly. The physician described the woman as "noncompliant" and "resistant" to taking her blood pressure medication as she had been directed, and he was clearly exasperated about her seeming unwillingness to follow his directions. The physician was clearly focusing on the "bottom line" of the patient's behavior—she was not doing what she was supposed to be doing.

The social worker, on the other hand, reacted to this woman's situation very differently. She raised questions about whether the patient had sufficient money to be able to afford to take the medication as she had been directed. Additionally, she wondered about the possible side effects and how these might have affected the patient's willingness to continue taking the medication as prescribed.

The physician clearly was concerned with a narrow focus on the woman's behavior; the social worker on the "bigger picture" of the forces that might be affecting that behavior: economic and value-related. One had "ruled out" dimensions of the problem; the other "ruled in" still other variables!

Emphasis on self-help and self-determination. In addition to representing the major influences of psychosocial factors in shaping health and assessing health problems, social workers have traditionally emphasized the rights of their patients to self-determination and have worked to increase their self-help skills.[24] The avoidance of labeling and "blaming the victim" have also been major themes in social work practice and the development of interventions. More recently, a renewed emphasis in social work has underscored the principle of patient self-determination and empowerment. This theme embodies a shift away from professionally determined problem definitions and solutions, toward consumer-defined needs and personal processes of discovering or creating ways of meeting them.[25]

Teamwork and value conflicts. Unlike other health professions, social work has a well-developed theme on the socialization of social workers in the collaborative or teamwork setting. For example, how social workers become socialized into a clinical team has been described as a process of successive role changes mediated by coaching from the instructor, the development of unique language for the team, and the growth in assertiveness skills.[26]

In addition to the acquisition of the values of patient autonomy and empowerment, social workers grapple with the value conflicts implicit in collaborative practice. For example, when interdisciplinary collaboration and patient advocacy—both important social work values—conflict, which should take precedence? Similarly, most codes of professional ethics have been developed for individual disciplines, but what happens when these come into conflict on the IHCT?[27] This dilemma is perhaps particularly compelling in social work, because this profession has traditionally been the one most associated with patient responsibility and self-determination.

Overall, the centrality of values and value conflicts seems to characterize the literature on socialization into social work. Reflection on value conflicts between social work and medicine, for example, is a constant theme, as are moral dilemmas in collaborative practice in general. The traditional knowledge, skills, and values emphasis in professional development is interpreted in the reverse order for social work, where it is recognized that values take precedence over knowledge.[28] Values are put at the very center of social work practice, with regard to both professional–professional interaction and professional–patient relationships. In this aspect, social work is unique in placing this aspect of clinical practice at the very core of what it means to be a professional.

The changing face of social work. Research by Netting and Williams[29] highlights the emerging "crisis" in social work as a profession, suggesting that it needs to redefine and clarify its role and its perception by other health professions, particularly medicine and nursing. This "problem" has been previously studied and characterized by other researchers.[30] In particular, in a case manager role context, nurses and physicians tend to downplay the importance of social work training, misunderstanding the background and educational preparation of social workers in general. Despite attempts to emphasize the uniqueness of social work, educators and practitioners in this profession must respond to the current forces in the health care system that tend to downplay the importance of social work and create the perception that other health care professionals, such as nurses, can easily pick up this role along with their own. This is a good example of how current forces in the health care system can continue shaping the identities of different health care professions.

IMPLICATIONS FOR CLINICAL PRACTICE: WHAT DIFFERENCES DO THESE VALUES MAKE?

These value differences acquired as an integral aspect of professional socialization make a major difference in patterns of clinical practice, affecting elements related to how practitioners define problems, grapple with issues defining quality of life, and practice collaboratively in decision making.

Defining the Problem: Clinical Assessment and Values

Every definition of a clinical problem consists of a factual and a value component. There is no purely "objective" basis for defining a problem in the absence of some value that is potentially affected by this "factual" state of affairs. Moreover, value orientations—as just discussed—can affect one's view of reality and the selection of information that one considers important to defining a problem in the first place. For example, as already mentioned, professionals may differ in their logic of clinical assessment— that is, how to define the problem. This difference may be characterized by two different styles of practice, one emphasizing ruling out problems by systematically eliminating possibilities until only one problem and a corresponding solution are discovered. In contrast, the other approach of ruling in problems relies on expanding the range of professional view to encompass an increasingly long list of potential factors.

For example, physicians—with their more reductionistic values—are trained in diagnostic techniques that narrow down the range of options, heavily relying on "objective" data such as laboratory tests in the process. Social workers, on the other hand, with their more holistic values are taught to go beyond the narrow presenting problem to incorporate larger psychosocial issues, such as income, family relationships, and the environment. In this process, they tend to rely on "subjective" data collected by interviews that are heavily interpreted by clinical judgment and experience. Nurses, depending on their background and training, may fall somewhere between these two extremes. Nurse practitioners tend to be more closely aligned with the biomedical model, whereas clinical nurse specialists have traditionally been considered more holistic in their approach to the patient.

Analyzing these value differences more closely, it is apparent that the traditional orientation of medicine toward the patient is to drown out his or her perspective in the process of making clinical assessments, virtually constructing the reality of the patient's condition through powerful medical imperatives to select only the "most important" information; to distance the practitioner from the patient; and otherwise to dehumanize, depersonalize, and decontextualize the patient in the interest of "objective" clinical judgment. Nursing in general and social work, on the other hand, have countervailing pressures to take on a real understanding of the "patient as person," to participate in the patient's world as a way of both understanding it and revealing their own humanity and, even, vulnerability. The approaches of nursing—excluding the more biomedical models of nursing—and social work are more inclusive and holistic than that of medicine.

This difference leads to a communication gap between professionals due to the differing assumptions about the importance of incorporating the patient's definition of the "problem" into the clinical assessment process. The communication problem here is that a major conceptual gap may exist between professionals and laypersons with regard to their construction of meaning of health and health-related problems. Providers and patients approach health issues from different perspectives—with the former reflecting the professional and organizational concepts and patterns of practice in which they have been trained, and the latter embodying different influences from their personal experiences, familial contexts, and cultural backgrounds.[31] Providers and patients speak different languages, although they may use the same words.

Moreover, because of differentials in power between the professional and the patient, the professional's definition of need, or the "problem" to be "solved," usually takes precedence over that of the patient. The person who controls the definition of the problem simultaneously defines the range of options available to solve it. In other words, recipients of clinical care must have genuine input into the basic construction of need and the concepts used to describe it, or else patients will be prevented from effective dialogue and discussion regarding the important outcomes of the needs assessment process.

Insofar as different health care professions are trained to emphasize or deemphasize the need for this patient input—depending on their values related to patient autonomy and control over the clinical decision-making process—these differences can be extremely important in distinguishing divergent styles of practice and, consequently, communication problems on IHCTs. Nowhere are these issues more apparent than in consideration of quality of life issues.

Quality of Life: Using the Same Words but with Different Meanings

The concept of *quality of life* means very different things to different people, whether providers or patients. In assessing these clinically significant differences, it is important that we carefully examine our thought and language, and ask the question: "Do we understand and communicate what we really mean?" In particular, personal, professional, and cultural values play an important role in defining and operationalizing the concept of quality of life. For example, a poor quality of life for one person may be a rich life for another: What we might consider to be a life full of sickness, frailty, and dependence might provide another person with new insights into the existential nature of human life and its continual conditionality and precariousness.[32] Importantly, overemphasis on individual independence in constructing a definition of quality of life may neglect the values of community, collectivism, and interdependence that are equally important in human existence.

Professionals, in particular, differ with regard to their definitions of quality of life—differences with important implications for their ability to communicate over issues affecting clinical decision making. For example, research in nursing homes has found that physicians and nursing assistants (whom we may consider to be aligned generally with nursing professional practice models) differ considerably on their feelings about the basis for life-extending treatment and the meaning of care.[33] To the nursing assistants, caring is a more important factor in quality of life than the mental and physical status of the patient; on the other hand, the treatability of a condition tends to be equated by the physicians with higher quality of life for the patient. Differing interpretations of the concept of quality of life underlie these differences in approaches to care. For most physicians, quality of life is related to mental status or freedom from mental impairment; by contrast, quality of life for nurses is more relative. Physical strength, even in the presence of mental impairment, is considered a key determinant of life quality. By contrast, social workers consider the ability of patients to live where they want to be a major factor in quality of life.

These differences in defining quality of life may be understood within the larger framework of disparities in the perceptions of ethical problems by physicians and nurses. Divergence between these two professions with regard to the recognition of moral dilemmas in practice suggests that such differences are crucial to understanding why communication about value-laden concepts can be so difficult. For example, although physicians and nurses have been found to differ significantly within each of their respective professional groups with regard to how often they perceive ethical dilemmas, nurses more often report conflicts with physicians over ethical dilemmas than are physicians to recognize disagreements with nurses.[34]

Other research has also found significant differences between nurses and physicans with regard to the ethical problems they identify.[35] For example, three quarters of the problems centering on a patient's quality of life were described by physicians rather than nurses. This disagreement over ethics problems is seen as a function of professional orientation and socialization, with nurses increasingly oriented toward patient-centered issues—such as patient preferences, family issues, pain control, implementing treatments, and discharge planning. By contrast, physicians are directed more toward problems embodying increased concern about the cost of care and the proper use of medical resources—such as quality of life, economic factors, and inappropriate admissions. Importantly, these physicians' concerns about quality of life are consistent with previous research linking life-quality considerations to decisions to withhold therapy, and to the tendency of physicians to rate the life quality of chronically ill elderly more negatively than do their patients.

In addition to medicine and nursing, social work offers another perspective on the differences underlying the health professions regarding life-quality interpretations. As explored earlier, social work has traditionally represented the broader psychosocial perspective on quality of life concerns in health and illness. This view entails the involvement of several relevant dimensions, including: (a) an assessment of the social environment (including family, social support, economic and cultural factors, and the physical setting), (b) the right of the individual to make his or her own decisions (autonomy), (c) the identification and mobilization of resources in the family and the community, and (d) mediation among the major professional and institutional "players" in defining and solving the individual's "problem.[36] This philosophical orientation ensures that the perspective of the individual on quality of life will be incorporated into the ongoing clinical discussion among the other health professionals on the team, the patient, and the social worker.

Values and Collaborative Practice

Insofar as collaborative practice models will become increasingly important in the delivery of health care in the future, it is essential that health care professionals acquire new appreciation for both the knowledge and skills needed on IHCTs and, perhaps more importantly, for the values represented by interdisciplinary teamwork. Interdisciplinary conflicts have been described for nurse-physician interactions,[37] social worker–physician relationships,[38] and nurse-social worker collaboration.[39] Although these have traditionally been couched in terms of role conflict—based on the conceptualization of professional socialization as the acquisition of specific roles—another, more useful way would be as value conflict. Additionally, the preferred styles of interaction of health care professionals may change when they are in conflict. One study found that under normal circumstances, the interaction patterns of nurses and social workers were most alike (nurturing). However, under conditions of conflict, the interaction patterns of physicians and nurses were most alike (avoiding).[40]

Additionally, conflicts may exist between professionals based on their value orientation to the patient. For example, social workers' ability to communicate on the interprofessional team may be impaired by their socialization and professional orientation.[41] Their lack of training in the more biomedical basis of health care can be a problem when discussing specific cases with physicians and nurses. Given the central importance of including in clinical decision-making processes individuals' values and personal perspectives on what constitutes quality of life for them, it seems imperative that this essential orientation not be lost in the dialogue among the different professions represented on the IHCT.

For health profession educators, the question now becomes one of how to promote the development of greater appreciation for the sounds of different perspectives or voices on IHCTs and increased recognition of the fact that absent voices really do make a difference in the quality of care.[42] Far from being rigid roles into which professionals have been socialized and trained, these values or voices represent unique views of the self and the patient—as well as other professionals—that are the products of a complex interaction between themselves and their colleagues, the larger institutional environment, and their patients. In this process, the distinction between themselves as professionals and as persons may become blurred, because they have internalized the very values essential to their modes of practice.

Thus, it is essential that professionals learn to recognize and appreciate that each has a different voice—a perspective or way of "being in the clinical world"—that is equally valid and valued. Perhaps most importantly, it is the voice of the patient that is the most critical and that must increasingly be seen as the core essence guiding professional practice. The metaphor of the "reflective practitioner" has been proposed for one who develops an appreciation for those "gray areas" of clinical practice where value conflicts and moral dilemmas are encountered, where the true artistry of professional practice is evident. Perhaps we need to develop an auditory metaphor in addition to this cognitive one: the reflective practitioner is also the "hearing practitioner," who is a good listener and whose own voice does not drown out the voices of other professionals or the patient. Similarly, however, there may be times when an individual professional's voice should be raised in a leadership role to provide guidance for the rest of the health care team, much as a vocalist takes the lead in a musical performance, with the chorus taking a background and supportive role.

SUMMARY

In summary, we need to train health care professionals to both reflect on, and listen to, the values and voices of others. "Listening with the inner ear" to what is being said in professional–professional and professional–patient communication becomes the basis for acquiring professional judgment in collaborative practice settings. This goal can be accomplished if we first recognize the limitations of the ways in which we currently train health care providers by isolating them from the worlds of each other and the patient. Then, we need to develop opportunities for practicing the essential skills in listening to oneself and to others. These opportunities should be provided for both health professions students and currently practicing professionals, who may have had little—if any—formal orientation to teamwork or collaborative practice.

We now have the theoretical foundation for how to do this, and some specific suggestions to follow. The challenge lies in implementing this new vision in the educational and clinical contexts where we train both health sciences students and practicing health care professionals.

NOTES

1. McClelland, M., & Sands, R. G. (1993). The missing voice in interdisciplinary communication. *Qualitative Health Research, 3*, 74–90.

2. Gilligan, C. (1982*). In a different voice: Psychological theory and women's development.* Cambridge, MA: Harvard University Press.

3. Clark, P. G. (1996). Communication between provider and patient: Values, biography, and empowerment in clinical practice. *Ageing and Society, 16*, 747–774.

4. Kaufman, S. R. (1986). *The ageless self: Sources of meaning in late life.* Madison: University of Wisconsin Press, p. 24.

5. Ford, C. V. (1983). *The somatizing disorders: Illness as a way of life.* New York: Elsevier Science Publications.

6. Schön, D. A. (1987). *Educating the reflective practitioner.* San Francisco, CA: Jossey-Bass.

7. Kaufman, S. R. (1995). Decision making, responsibility, and advocacy in geriatric medicine: Physician dilemmas with elderly in the community. *The Gerontologist, 35,* 481–488.

8. Bloom, S. W. (1979). Socialization for the physician's role: A review of some contributions of research to theory. In E. C. Shapiro & L. M. Lowenstein (Eds.), *Becoming a physician: Development of values and attitudes in medicine* (pp. 3–52). Cambridge, MA: Ballinger; Bloom, S. W. (1989). The medical school as social organization: The sources of resistance to change. *Medical Education, 23,* 228–241.

9. See, for example, Davidson, W.A.S. (1991). Metaphors of health and aging: Geriatrics as metaphor. In G. M. Kenyon, J. E. Birren, & J.J.F. Schroots (Eds.), *Metaphors of aging in science and the humanities* (pp. 173–184). New York: Springer; Reiser, S. J. (1993). The era of the patient: Using the experience of illness in shaping the missions of health care. *Journal of the American Medical Association, 269,* 1012–1017; Risse, G. B. (1982). Once on top, now on tap: American physicians view their relationships with patients, 1920–1970. In G. J. Agich (Ed.), *Responsibility in health care* (pp. 23–49). Dordrecht, Holland: D. Reidel; Roter, D. L., & Hall, J. A. (1992). *Doctors talking with patients/patients talking with doctors.* Westport, CT: Auburn House.

10. Furnham, A. (1988). Values and vocational choice: A study of value differences in medical, nursing, and psychology students. *Social Science and Medicine, 26,* 613–618; Geller, G., Faden, R. R., & Levine, D. M. (1990). Tolerance for ambiguity among medical students: Implications for their selection, training, and practice. *Social Science and Medicine, 31,* 619–624.

11. Fasano, L. A., Muskin, P. R., & Sloan, R. P. (1993). The impact of medical education on students' perceptions of patients. *Academic Medicine, 68* (Suppl.), S43–S45.

12. Ford, *The somatizing disorders.*

13. Self, D. J., Schrader, D. E., Baldwin, D. C., & Wolinsky, F. D. (1991). A pilot study of the relationship of medical education and moral development. *Academic Medicine, 66,* 629.

14. Andre, J. (1992). Learning to see: Moral growth during medical training. *Journal of Medical Ethics, 18,* 148–152.

15. Mizrahi, T. (1984). Managing medical mistakes: Ideology, insularity and accountability among internists-in-training. *Social Science and Medicine, 19,* 135–146.

16. Mizrahi, T. (1986). *Getting rid of patients: Contradictions in the socialization of physicians.* New Brunswick, NJ: Rutgers University Press.

17. Roter & Hall, *Doctors talking with patients/patients talking with doctors.*

18. Mishler, E. G. (1984). *The discourse of medicine: Dialectics of medical interviews.* Norwood, NJ: Ablex.

19. Fagermoen, M. S. (1995). *The meaning of nurses' work: A descriptive study of values fundamental to professional identity in nursing.* Unpublished doctoral dissertation, the University of Rhode Island, Kingston.

20. Seed, A. (1994). Patients to people. *Journal of Advanced Nursing, 19,* 738–748.

21. See Parse, R. R. (1987). *Nursing science: Major paradigms, theories, and critiques.* Philadelphia: W. B. Saunders; Parse, R. R. (1992). Human becoming: Parse's theory of nursing. *Nursing Science Quarterly, 5,* 35–42.

22. Mizrahi, T., & Abramson, J. (1985). Sources of strain between physicians and social workers: Implications for social workers in health care settings. *Social Work in Health Care, 10*(3), 33–51.

23. Qualls, S. H., & Czirr, R. (1988). Geriatric health teams: Classifying models of professional and team functioning. *The Gerontologist, 28,* 372–376.

24. Kane, R. A. (1975). *Interprofessional teamwork* (Manpower monograph No. 8). Syracuse, NY: Syracuse University School of Social Work.

25. DeJong, G. (1984). Independent living: From social movement to analytic paradigm. In P. Marinelli & A. Dell (Eds.), *The psychological and social impact of physical disability* (pp. 39–64). New York: Springer; Tower, K. D. (1994). Consumer-centered social work practice: Restoring client self-determination. *Social Work, 39,* 191–196.

26. Sands, R. G. (1989). The social worker joins the team: A look at the socialization process. *Social Work in Health Care, 14*(2), 1–14.

27. Abramson, M. (1984). Collective responsibility in interdisciplinary collaboration: An ethical perspective for social workers. *Social Work in Health Care, 10*(1), 35–43; Mailick, M. D., & Ashley A. A. (1981). Politics of interprofessional collaboration: Challenge to advocacy. *Social Casework, 62,* 131–137.

28. Mizrahi & Abramson, "Sources of strain."

29. Netting, F. E., & Williams, F. G. (1996). Case manager–physician collaboration: Implications for professional identity, roles, and relationships. *Health and Social Work, 21,* 216–224; Netting, F. E., & Williams, F. G. (1997, March). *Preparing the next generation of geriatric social workers to collaborate with primary care physicians.* Paper presented at the annual meeting of the Council on Social Work Education, Chicago, IL.

30. Williams, R. A., & Williams, C. C. (1982). Hospital social workers and nurses: Interprofessional perceptions and experiences. *Journal of Nursing Education, 21*(5), 16–21.

31. Dill, A. (1993). Defining needs, defining systems: A critical analysis. *The Gerontologist, 33,* 453–460.

32. Gadow, S. (1983). Frailty and strength: The dialectic in aging. *The Gerontologist, 23,* 144–147.

33. Kayser-Jones, J. S. (1986). Distributive justice and the treatment of acute illness in nursing homes. *Social Science in Medicine, 23,* 1279–1286.

34. Gramelspacher, G. P., Howell, J. D., & Young, M. J. (1986). Perceptions of ethical problems by nurses and doctors. *Archives of Internal Medicine, 146,* 577–578.

35. Walker, R. M., Miles, S. H., Stocking, C. B., & Siegler, M. (1991). Physicians' and nurses' perceptions of ethics problems on general medical services. *Journal of General Internal Medicine, 6,* 424–429.

36. Jones, J. M., Meredith, S., Wadas, L., Watt, S., & Weisz, E. (1991). The contribution and role of the social worker. In National Advisory Council on Aging (Ed.), *Geriatric assessment and treatment: Members of the team* (pp. 35–52). Ottawa, ON: Minister of Supply and Services Canada.

37. Stein, L. I. (1967). The doctor-nurse game. *Archives of General Psychiatry, 16,* 699–703; Stein, L. I., Watts, D. T., & Howell, T. (1990). The doctor-nurse game revisited. *The New England Journal of Medicine, 322,* 546–549; Watts, D. T., McCaulley, B. L., & Priefer, B. A. (1990). Physician-nurse conflict: Lessons from a clinical experience. *Journal of the American Geriatrics Society, 38,* 1151–1152.

38. Mizrahi, T., & Abramson, J. (1985). Sources of strain between physicians and social workers: Implications for social workers in health care settings. *Social Work in Health Care, 10*(3), 33–51.

39. Lowe, J. I., & Herranen, M. (1978). Conflict in teamwork: Understanding roles and relationships. *Social Work in Health Care, 3,* 323–330; Lowe, J. I., & Herranen, M. (1981). Understanding teamwork: Another look at the concepts. *Social Work in Health Care, 7*(2), 1–11.

40. Drinka, T.J.K., Miller, T. F., & Goodman, B. M. (1996). Characterizing motivational styles of professionals who work on interdisciplinary healthcare teams. *Journal of Interprofessional Care, 10,* 51–61.

41. Kane, *Interprofessional teamwork.*

42. Aumann, G.M.-E., & Cole, T. R. (1991). In whose voice? Composing a lifesong collaboratively. *The Journal of Clinical Ethics, 2,* 45–49; McClelland & Sands, The missing voice.

5

The Science and the Art of Interdisciplinary Practice

Becoming a member of an IHCT should change a person, both in terms of overt behavior and with respect to the way the person thinks about his or her work. This change may be considered an aspect of what is meant when one becomes a "team player" and not just a "team member." This transformation is a developmental process that progresses through stages, although individuals may advance, regress, and stagnate at different levels at different times. In other words, teamwork is really team work that requires an active engagement on the part of both the individual member and the group as a whole. Passivity is not a virtue when it comes to the kind of commitment and dedication needed to become a member of an effective IHCT!

The goal of developing an effective health care team is often viewed primarily as a group process issue: How the team evolves and develops as a small group with respect to such issues as member roles, trust, and shared norms becomes the focus. Indeed, much of the literature on teams is based on research into various stages of team development. Although this is certainly an important aspect of the evolution of a team, it is only one way of understanding the kind of transformation that occurs—and at the level of the group or collective. However, a clinical team is much more than the simple sum of individuals working together as a group: It is a complex entity of providers who are trained in different fields or professions, and who use different tools, frameworks, and approaches to the patient. As the team develops more experience in working together, transformations occur within members that reflect an internal change in the thought processes and normative assumptions on which they base their behavior and practice. These changes are the focus of this chapter.

An insight into these transformations may be gained by re-examining the metaphor of the "reflective practitioner." Remember that the reflective practitioner is one skilled not only in the scientific or technical aspects of the profession, but also in the more artistic dimensions that deal with value dilemmas and conflicts—where the precise course of action is unclear because of competing values that lead in different directions. Overemphasis on the technical aspects of one's profession can lead to a situation that may be called the "unreflective practitioner." This individual is on "auto pilot" in his or her daily clinical work and does not recognize or deal effectively with the gray areas of practice where the limits of knowledge are reached. Recognizing that all knowledge is limited; that it is by its very nature imperfect, partial, and incomplete; and that simple knowledge is not sufficient to get the professional "off the hook" in dealing with ethical dilemmas in practice—these are the characteristics of the reflective practitioner. As Kaufman[1] suggested in the area of geriatric practice, particularly dilemmatic are those areas in which the precise course of action to be taken is not clear. This lack of clarity is due to conflicts between competing values that underlie different courses of action. Indeed, as she argued, geriatric practice is by its very nature bound up in moral ambiguity in which clinical decision making is inextricably tied to questions of "what to do?" and "how to act?" that are moral in nature.

It is our contention that team practice in general and effective teamwork in particular are based on two "foundations of understanding" among the team members suggested by this metaphor of the reflective practitioner (i.e., "cognitive maps" and "value maps"). Cognitive maps embody members' understanding of how they and different professions on the team use the knowledge they have mastered as a part of their profession, and also recognize its limitations. Value maps suggest that they must also understand how the different values and value orientations of the team's members affect how they grapple with the significant ethical issues encountered in clinical practice. These insights develop as the team evolves, and their level of attainment may be considered a marker of team development.

COGNITIVE MAPS: THE KNOWLEDGE AND SKILLS BASE

The health care professions are based on the mastery of, and the ability to generate and utilize, specific types of complex information. Each discipline or profession has a unique approach to understanding and using this information; indeed, the power of a profession is based in large part on its understanding and use of this specific knowledge base. Professions have developed historically as they have increasingly defined and defended the specific nature and application of this information. The knowledge and skills base underlying a particular profession has been termed its *cognitive map,* representing the entire paradigmatic and conceptual apparatus used by a discipline and including its basic concepts, modes of inquiry, problem definitions, observational categories, representational techniques, standards of proof, types of explanation, and general ideas of what represents a discipline.[2]

Why is an understanding of cognitive maps important in IHCTs? If members of a team do not possess at least a basic understanding of each other's cognitive maps, it is likely that misunderstandings will result. The comments or suggestions of one team member will be mentally processed and understood in terms of the others' respective cognitive maps. Under these circumstances, it is possible for team members from different disciplines to look at the same thing but not see the same thing. We often use slides of ambiguous figures to illustrate this point in a workshop presentation—the kinds of figures in which some see faces, others a vase; some a duck, others a rabbit.

Consider also the following IHCT example: The term *assessment* is used by most health professions, but it can have very different meanings across the discipines of medicine, nursing, and social work. Physicians tend to focus on a more limited range of issues related to a specific disease process in a particular organ system, whereas nursing focuses more holistically on the individual. Social work widens the perspective to capture the broader social, environmental, and economic contexts. Moreover, how the patient's "problem" is framed at the time of the initial assessment will determine the range of potential solutions to it—such is the power wielded in "problem defining" or assessing activities.

The Case of the "Constipation Caper" and Cognitive Maps

A pharmacy student on an interdisciplinary health promotion team at a university was participating in a discussion during a group workshop on health issues at a local senior housing site. An older woman who was a participant confided in him that she had been having trouble with constipation and asked him for some advice on what to do.

The pharmacy student's immediate response and recommendation was for her to ask her physican for a prescription for a stool softener or laxative, or to consider an over-the-counter option at her local pharmacy. He clearly was responding to her question based on his pharmaceutical profession's cognitive map.

Overhearing this exchange was another member of the health promotion team, a nursing student. She immediately spoke up and said, "You don't have to take a pill!" Instead, she suggested that the older woman could solve this problem by drinking at least eight glasses of water a day, getting more exercise, and eating foods high in fiber.

The pharmacy student was speechless for a moment (you could see his jaw drop!), and then he blurted out that he had never even thought of these approaches to her problem. Suddenly, the "light bulb" came on in his head as he realized how different health professions approach problems and their solutions differently, all based on varying cognitive maps.

Members of IHCTs must openly communicate with each other in order for them to incorporate the cognitive maps of others into their own framing of "what is the problem" and "how it can be solved." For example, eliminating the use of jargon is an important first step. We have sat in on team meetings that we have had to interrupt to ask the speaker to "please explain that term" that no one else understood. Similarly, the use of metaphors to describe the different roles or approaches of different professions may be helpful: the doctor as "detective," the nurse as "educator," and the social worker as "advocate" are images that come to mind.

VALUE MAPS: THE NORMATIVE BASIS OF A PROFESSION

Understanding information and knowledge is only a part of what constitutes a profession, however. Equally important, we argue, are the less quantifiable dimensions of practice, which we discuss under the rubric of *values*. These fall within Schön's domain of the art of professional practice, as contrasted with the science. This skill constitutes the ability of a practitioner to grapple with the value conflicts and moral dilemmas that characterize professionalism. It is also related to the intellectual and factual basis of practice, as intellectual and ethical development have been shown to be interrelated.[3] Our approach to factual information is contingent on our personal and professional value orientations.[4]

As explored in the previous chapter, different health care professions are based on different values and value systems. Health care providers are socialized and acculturated into these value systems as a part of their professional education and training. It is only when they are thrust into an interdisciplinary experience or setting that they realize these values vary across the different health disciplines—an insight that is fostered by interdisciplinary education and clinical practice programs. By recognizing that different professions have different value maps—the basic ethical principles that guide practice, modes of moral reasoning, and methods to deal with conflicts among competing principles—health care providers begin to realize that these differences reveal significant information about the origin and nature of their responsibilities toward others—including other professionals as well as the patient.

Value Maps on a Health Care Team

A physician and a social worker on an interdisciplinary community clinic-based assessment team were discussing the case of an elderly gentleman living alone in his own home. The clinic had been called earlier in the week by a neighbor of the man, who was concerned about his well-being.

When she paid a visit to the elderly man, the social worker was appalled at his poor living conditions—his house was filled with cats and piles of old newspapers—but he seemed lucid and fully capable of making decisions for himself. He told the social worker that he did not want to "go on welfare" and that he was happy living the way he was. He did not want or need anything, thank you very much.

When the social worker presented her findings the next day at the team meeting, the physician on the team suggested that this man could really benefit from a medical work-up, and that the team should somehow arrange for him to be "dragged in" if need be for a comprehensive assessment "for his own good." The physician also suggested that they clean up his house so that it would be a safer place in which to live.

The social worker's response to the physician was that this elderly man was totally capable of choosing how he wanted to live, based on respect for his autonomy. For her, the value of his autonomy was the most important value, even if it meant that he might be putting himself at risk for injury.

For the physician, however, it was apparent that the value of professional beneficence—doing good—overrode his concern about the man's ability and right to make his own decisions, even ones that others might consider to be bad, misinformed, or risky.

Hopefully, members of an IHCT come to recognize the important advantage—the value—that collaborative work and problem solving have to offer. The value of teamwork itself comes to displace the model of the "unidisciplinary" practitioner into which the providers were originally socialized in their respective professional programs. Rather than subscribing to the highly individualistic professional norm that many health care settings reinforce, team members begin to appreciate the distinct advantages of cooperation and collaboration. In this sense, interdependence displaces independence and leads to the recognition of the limits of each profession when dealing with multifaceted health problems.

Levels of Values

We may also conceptualize the transformation in values that occurs in the process of becoming an IHCT as a dynamic interplay among four different levels of value-based loyalties or responsibilities of team members. These levels mirror to some extent the evolution of health care professions to higher levels of organizational complexity:

Personal level. The health care professional has an interpersonal relationship with the individual patient, guided by certain norms, principles, and responsibilities that are reflective of the individual provider. The provider has a personal responsibility for the welfare and well-being of the patient. Much of traditional biomedical ethics focuses on this level.

Professional level. Personal responsibility remains important, but now it is bolstered by the norms and practice standards of different professional associations—such as those for medicine, nursing, and social work—all of which have ethical codes and guidelines.

Teamwork level. Emerging during the course of team development is a growing sense of loyalty to the shared norms and principles of the team, and to the very concept of teamwork itself. At this level, different members of the team still retain their own personal and professional guides for conduct, but superimposed on them are new team-based principles that may even bring members into conflict with their own or their profession's precepts.

Organizational level. Increasingly, organizations and their values wield significant power in health care decision making. Managed care organizations, for example, may emphasize economic values in their attempts to control provider behavior and affect established professional norms. Provider conduct, performance, and clinical outcomes are increasingly scrutinized with regard to cost. Importantly, these values and forces come from professionals (such as managers) outside of the traditional health care decision-making context.

These four levels exist simultaneously on IHCTs, and they do so in a dynamic tension in which they may reinforce or conflict with each other. This situation gives new meaning to the concept of the "reflective practitioner"—professionals must now become aware of the gray areas of ethical conflict in their own domain of practice, as well as that of the clinical team on which they serve. As discussed in chapter 4, the value orientations of different health professions—their unique "voices" or ways of being in the world—may conflict, and this conflict will have to be resolved if the team is to continue to work effectively together.

Value Conflict on a Team

A social worker member of a hospital-based assessment team was interviewing a patient to gather the psychosocial information necessary for her participation in the next day's team conference.

The patient revealed some very personal information about his background to the social worker and asked that she keep this information confidential. She did not know how to respond to the patient: on the one hand, she wanted to agree to this request, based on her personal and professional obligation to respect the confidentiality of patient information. On the other hand, the team was based on the open sharing of information that its members gained about the patients it was assessing and for whom it was developing care plans.

The social worker was caught in a dilemma created at the interface of differing levels of responsibility.

TEAM DEVELOPMENT AND COGNITIVE AND NORMATIVE TRANSFORMATION

An insight into the potential transformations in the cognitive and normative bases of professional practice achieved through participation on IHCTs can be gained by examining the research into college student development—specifically the work of Perry.[5] Perry postulated that students move through four stages in their understanding of knowledge and values: dualism, multiplicity, relativism, and commitment in relativism. Although based on research with a population different from health care professionals, nevertheless the results are suggestive of a way of thinking about similar changes in team members. These changes may occur as they deal with the challenges encountered in interdisciplinary settings, where they are confronted with very different ways of clinical understanding and acting.

Dualism

At this stage, a person believes that knowledge is simply the accumulation of facts: The more facts you know, the smarter you are. Authority figures—such as parents and professors—have the "answers," which are simple and definitive. The world is divided into those who know and those who do not; those who agree with them are good and right; those who disagree are bad and wrong.

Multiplicity

At this level, there is beginning to be an awareness that ambiguity exists in some areas of knowledge, but this may be due to personal factors (e.g., a professor's ignorance) or just to the state of research into a specific issue.

An individual at this stage may come to feel that because there are no clearly "right" answers in a particular field, anyone can think anything.

Relativism

A person at this stage recognizes that ambiguity exists as a fact of life; all facts and theories are human constructs, and hence fallible. However, one can still create theories that help us to organize knowledge and understand what we observe and how we should act. It is important to be balanced and consider different points of view. Experts are people who have more experience in this process and a wider "factual" base on which to draw.

Commitment in Relativism

A person at this stage has deliberately chosen, on reflection, to adhere to a particular school of thought or to stand up for a particular value. Other perspectives are seen as having validity, and the effective advocate of a particular position should be able to articulate his or her viewpoint and support it with evidence and sound reasoning.

Members of an IHCT may go through these stages at a level higher than that dealing specifically with the understanding of their own discipline's knowledge base. Entering the team experience forces them to go beyond their perception of the supremacy of their own discipline ("I'm right and you're wrong") in approaching the patient; to a recognition of the existence of other approaches to dealing with problems; and finally to an understanding of how their particular approach differs from, yet may be similar to or complement, the others represented on the team. At this point, the team member may be able to make a commitment, perhaps for the first time, to what his or her own profession really means and represents. In parallel with this development of professional identity, a growing self-awareness comes with the recognition of the complexity of the professional world and the need to take possession of one's own, unique way of acting in it.

In our experience, students in particular enter an interdisciplinary team setting with a certain amount of ambivalence. In many cases, they have just barely mastered the professional knowledge base and values of their own profession, and now they are being challenged to reflect on these in the confusing context of other, sometimes conflicting, orientations. The result is that they move from a dualistic stage, in which they see value distinctions as right versus wrong within their respective disciplines, to an understanding of the multiplicity of values that characterize a range of professions. Ultimately, they are able to defend their own values in the context of an understanding of the values of others, the stage of commitment in relativism. The depth of real understanding of their own values comes from a recognition of the diversity that exists, a recognition that is made possible by the interprofessional experience—but with a new sense of affirmation that comes from having to grapple with the questions of who they are and what professional values they represent.

Identity Development on an IHCT

In a team-building course with which we have been associated, a student commented in her end-of-the-semester final project evaluation, "I [am] amazed to see how much I have changed over the semester. I am more confident in my role as a dietitian, and have increased my sense of security [in] being an active member of this team. I feel the personal attention I have received . . . and the team has helped to contribute to the positive behavior changes that I have encountered."

This transformation occurs not only vis-à-vis the other health professions, but also with respect to the patient. The focus of some of our educational team-building experiences has been on empowering patients to accept more accountability for their own health behavior and care. This team "mission" causes the students to reflect, in some cases for the first time, on how their own levels of professionalism may stand in the way of patients assuming more responsibility for their own health. They eventually come to recognize the need to form a partnership with the patient, rather than to assume they know what is best for him or her, thereby imposing their own values on defining the patient's problem and offering solutions to it. This insight grows out of a recognition of the need for health care professionals to respect patient autonomy, even when the professional paternalistically feels that he or she knows "what is best." This insight is incorporated into the previously discussed concept of the "reflective practitioner."

GAUGING COGNITIVE AND NORMATIVE CHANGES ON TEAMS

An essential aspect of learning about IHCTs is allowing students or trainees to reflect at the end of a workshop or semester on what they have learned. In our experience, this learning is often linked to the kinds of cognitive and normative changes just described. For example, we have had experience working with health professions students in a semester-long field experiential learning course on teamwork. Undergraduate and graduate students from nursing, pharmacy, dietetics, dental hygiene, and psychology participated in a weekly class seminar or discussion on topics relevant to

IHCTs. Additionally, they engaged in a fieldwork component that required the students to design, develop, and deliver a series of six to eight health promotion workshops to a group of community-dwelling older adults at a senior housing project site. The students were responsible for participant recruitment, assessment of needs for health-related information, topic selection, and the design of an appropriate curriculum. The fieldwork was done collaboratively, with students working in teams of four to six members, embodying a mix of health professions.

The students were required to write a final project description at the end of the semester, in addition to keeping a weekly journal that is described in more detail in chapter 8. The final project statement was an opportunity for them to look back over the course of the semester and to reflect on how they had changed personally and professionally. Excerpts from these reports, printed here, highlight the importance of changing cognitive and normative assumptions and orientations about what it means to be a health professional and the limits of their own knowledge when dealing with complex issues and problems.

Interdisciplinary Team Course: Summary Statements from Final Student Reports

Dietetics student (undergraduate). I would like to comment that I am grateful to have had this experience, and I am now a different person for this. In retrospect, it is amazing to look back to the first day of class when I was afraid to even talk because I thought I had nothing relevant to offer. Also, I felt intimidated by the fact that this was a graduate course, which consisted of a registered nurse and pharmacist as two of its members. Then there was me, an undergraduate in dietetics, who never worked with other disciplines before, and felt out of place from my usual class setting with all familiar faces. . . . Gradually, I realized we were all part of this "team" together, and we all had a common goal of patient welfare, which was the main force that united me to the other team members. Nobody really looked at me differently, and it was in my head that the rest of the team was better than me. It was not too long before I understood, that each discipline had a unique body of information to offer, and when all the members work together, the goal of patient welfare can be reached.

I am much more confident in my role as a dietitian and how I fit into the health care setting among other disciplines. Also, I am now aware of how I can still play an active role in delivering workshops with topics that do not directly relate to me. Furthermore, the black-and-white views I used to hold are now blending into a gray area that covers a much broader range of ideas and concepts, that I used to be too narrow minded to see. Now, there is a whole new world to explore, that I have missed out on in the past.

I now have a more open mind toward other disciplines, after I was convinced the team saw me as an equal. . . . Also, I have always been a person to take all the responsibilities on myself; I know that I will perform 110%, and have never heavily relied on others for help. Now, however, I do not have to carry that burden all on myself because I am limiting the knowledge passed on to my audience and I am wearing myself down. Learning to trust other members was probably the most difficult task to master.

Psychology student (undergraduate). The next conflict was at the workshop organizational meeting. In discussing the need to have a workshop on vitamins, [the dietetics student] felt unsure of her role as a dietitian discussing vitamins when she felt strongly against them as a dietary supplement. This conflict was resolved with clear communication and collaboration from the whole team, including [the student]. Our team was visibly maturing.

Pharmacy student 1 (undergraduate). I came to realize that conflict is not necessarily bad but a needed part of the learning process. It can be dealt with by looking at it as a challenge. Dealing with stressors and obstacles may make things more difficult initially but the end result is usually better. With the vitamin workshop [the dietetics student] and I had two different views but we were able to talk it out and mesh our ideas together. It took more effort but the resulting workshop was better and more practical for those involved than either of us could have done on our own.

Nursing student (graduate). Although I am greatly embarrassed to admit to it, I felt that I had a very good handle on interdisciplinary team dynamics. Now I have come to understand over the last 3 months that I had only the most rudimentary understanding of such principles that we have experienced during the semester. I had never understood the differences in multidisciplinary and interdisciplinary teams. I have begun to understand the greater benefits and efficiency that an interdisciplinary team can expect.

I have, through this semester, realized the strengths of other disciplines and therefore the limitations of my own experience and expertise. I have started requesting more input from some of the other disciplines both in the meeting and in the daily care for the patients in my care. There definitely is a more open line of communication between myself and other disciplines. I have finally grown to realize that no one professional has the answers to all of life's questions—especially when faced with the complex needs of the gerontological population. I also am in the process of becoming a more reflective practitioner in my nursing care. Sometimes there are no easy answers or solutions to dilemmas with health care situations. A reflective approach trains me in new ways of looking at situations I face daily.

Pharmacy student 2 (undergraduate). The journal allowed for a good amount of self-realization throughout the semester as our experiences were compiled on paper. This gave me a chance to look back and see how I have changed with regard to my views on the elderly population and the importance of the health care team—two positive changes that I have become very satisfied with.

As a "soon-to-be" professional, I have learned certain things about where I fit in on the team. I, being the pharmacist, will be the drug expert and should under no circumstances relinquish that role. There are, however, newfound roles that I have found available to assist on including physical assessment, patient education, and possibly some nutritional advice. Once I realized that very few professional boundaries are set in stone, I felt more integrated into the team and felt that I could contribute more.

[This course] has potentially done more for my career than any single course to date. The experiences that I have gained from this course will help to make me a better health care practitioner, educator, team member, and person. I have learned how to work well with others to achieve a set of goals as a unit, not individually; and also the confidence to fulfill my obligation to the team. It has also enabled me to have a chance to view the elderly in a different light than I am accustomed to, a welcomed opportunity.

In summary, these students reflect the internal, cognitive, and normative changes—directed both toward themselves and other health professions on the team—that we described as characteristics of the "reflective practitioner." The developmental process that led to these changes—and how to capture it—is described in more depth and detail in chapter 8.

METHODS TO PROMOTE COGNITIVE AND NORMATIVE DEVELOPMENT ON TEAMS

Emphasis on the theoretical underpinnings of IHCTs should not be interpreted to suggest that these concepts cannot be embodied in concrete methods to facilitate their understanding. For example, we have used journaling, case discussion, language and metaphor, and reflection time in furthering the acquisition of these insights by student and clinical practice teams.

Journaling

In team development courses and experiences, we have requested that trainees keep a detailed journal of their experience on the team, using a specified format that required a distinction among observational and theoretical or explanatory notes. This format forces the trainee to interpret or make meaning out of what has been experienced or observed. Because teamwork and team development are, at their core, experiential learning activities, keeping a journal has two distinct advantages. First, it is a record for trainees to "see how far they have come" from the beginning of the experience and thereby to reflect on their progress. Second, it represents an opportunity for the instructor or team trainer (who reads the journal) to "get inside" the individual's experience to understand the internal transformations in thinking, professional identity changes, and conflict both within the individual team member and between different team members. As such, the journal becomes a very important "window" for observing the development of the team members individually and as a group. The team trainer or instructor can then "coach" individual members or the group as a whole in the acquisition of the skills or behaviors necessary to move the team forward (the instructional metaphor of "coaching" and the use of journaling are explored in more detail in chapter 8).

Case Discussion

Clinical case studies are often written to be used in IHCT training settings, to illustrate the important reasons why more than one health care profession may be necessary to solve health-related problems, or to illustrate team dynamics and process issues—such as communication and conflict. Discussion of such cases—far from being used simply to come up with a "solution" to the clinical problem in as short a time as possible—provides an opportunity for exchanging disciplinary perspectives, learning the cognitive maps of other disciplines (as well as more fully understanding one's own), and sharing values that bear on assessing and seeking solutions to the problems represented in the case. The importance of involving and understanding the different distinct professional "voices" in the interdisciplinary team discussion can be highlighted.

Language and Metaphor

Special attention to the use and abuse of language is critical to the development of the IHCT. Some disciplines promote the use of specialized jargon to establish and reinforce professional barriers, giving one discipline power over another. Open communication demands that jargon be reduced or abolished, or else the team experience may collapse into an interdisciplinary Tower of Babel.

At the same time, the use of language to describe how different health care professions approach the patient, or solve problems, may reveal a significant amount about the use of information and the values underlying practice. For example, to some individuals the use of the words *patient* and *compliance* connote a passive involvement of an individual within a more medical model of care, whereas to others the use of terms such as *consumer* may suggest a more active, empowered role. Similarly, the phrase "placing the patient in a nursing home" carries with it a sense of depersonalization and objectification of a human being. Drawing attention to the use of language creates a fertile ground for understanding how professions see themselves and each other, as well as the patient, and thus it stimulates communication across disciplinary boundaries.

Also, as already discussed, the use of metaphor has been suggested as an excellent method to create cross-awareness of cognitive maps. This entails the development of verbal or visual analogies to assist in learning the observational categories of different disciplines. For example, for the physician, the metaphor "detective" may characterize his or her approach to the patient, emphasizing the importance of "clues" and assembling the pieces of the "puzzle" in differential diagnosis. Similarly, and in contrast, a nurse may be seen as a "facilitator" to help a patient understand the barriers standing in the way of more independent functioning in the face of an impairment. The emphasis in this facilitative role is more on the health professional as "educator" than as "detective."

The fact that different disciplines offer unique and powerful insights based on their own individual cognitive maps makes it essential for the team to make use of these perspectives, rather than to reduce all team activities to the level of the lowest common denominator of "common sense." The key becomes one of retaining and integrating these powerful methods while, at the same time, making the internal workings of each profession apparent and understandable in nontechnical language.

Reflection Time

Every IHCT needs time to reflect on how it is functioning as a team, rather than simply engaging in clinical, goal-directed, or problem-solving behavior. Time needs to be set aside on a regular basis for team maintenance issues relating to communication, conflict, roles, and troubleshooting. As in any relationship, time is required for celebrating successes and exploring the reasons for failures. In the crush to perform its mission, a team may find that the time available for such reflection is very limited, but it is essential that this time be set aside to deal with these issues. Otherwise, the existence of the team itself may be threatened, or its effectiveness and functioning severely impaired.

SUMMARY

In summary, becoming an IHCT "player" requires transformation both in one's personal viewpoint and in one's professional identity. This change may be conceptualized as occurring in cognitive and value maps, which are simply metaphors themselves for the types of internal "reprogramming" that goes along with becoming a member of an effective IHCT. In a sense, this discussion has highlighted these changes as goals rather than as inevitable outcomes of participating on an IHCT. As everyone who has participated on an IHCT knows, some team members do not go on to become team players (unfortunately). However, we hope that thinking of these changes in this way has made it more apparent what changes should occur and what types of goals we should set for teamwork training.

NOTES

1. Kaufman, S. R. (1995). Decision making, responsibility, and advocacy in geriatric medicine: Physician dilemmas with elderly in the community. *The Gerontologist, 35,* 481–488.

2. Petrie, H. G. (1976). Do you see what I see? The epistemology of interdisciplinary inquiry. *Journal of Aesthetic Education, 10,* 29–43.

3. Perry, W. G. (1970). *Forms of intellectual and ethical development in the college years: A scheme.* New York: Holt, Rinehart & Winston.

4. Potter, R. B. (1969). *War and moral discourse.* Richmond, VA: John Knox Press.

5. Perry, *Forms of intellectual and ethical development.*

6

Leadership and Power for
Interdisciplinary Practice

Chapter 1 introduced a team that was being faced with major changes in clinic operations. Some team members, like the physician, wanted to accept the decision of management about efficient and inefficient clinics. Other team members, like the nurse and social worker, wanted to be more proactive and to meet with management about this issue. We can speculate about who the leaders were in this case. However, it is more interesting to consider who should have been the leaders. The physician appeared to be the team leader because the administrator had summoned him as team representative. The physician also seemed to have a lot of influence with the team because when he suggested that the team accept the administrator's decision and stop meeting to discuss difficult cases, many of the team members appeared to comply. Perhaps the nurse practitioner and social worker would have exercised interdisciplinary leadership if they had gone to the administrator. However, if other team members did not accept the nurse practitioner and social worker in that role, their leadership would have been much less certain. These are some of the complexities and uncertainties of interdisciplinary leadership.

Thus far, we have seen that IHCTs provide a forum for health care providers to address complex issues in patient care. Complex problems have many causes and effects that are initially unknown. Uncovering and addressing these related issues takes different kinds of leadership assumed by those who have the skills to define and address the underlying problems. Volumes have been written about leadership, and yet its essence remains largely misunderstood. We understand interdisciplinary leadership even less as it has been researched very little. In fact, there is no widely accepted term for the kind of leadership that is discussed in this chapter. Interdisciplinary leadership must take place in a way that allows health professionals to work across disciplinary boundaries. Interdisciplinary leadership can be formal, informal, or both. However, the concept of interdisciplinary leadership is complex and even when it is understood it may not be allowed or encouraged.

BACKGROUND FOR INTERDISCIPLINARY LEADERSHIP

Organizational models and metaphors have shaped and will continue to shape the way that leadership is viewed in business organizations.[1] These models and metaphors refer to structural, behavioral, political, and cultural processes and are increasingly shaping leadership in health care organizations in general and IHCTs in particular as more health care organizations are led by those trained in schools of management. Structural and behavioral characteristics are dominant in these models and metaphors.

Some of these models and metaphors are more favorable to interdisciplinary leadership than others. Structural models contend that leadership roles and functions in organizations are assigned and deliberate and that power is unevenly distributed.[2] An opposing behaviorist or humanist view suggests that the equalization of power in organizations is essential[3] and that the equalization of power is basic to modern organizational development.[4] Leadership under the humanist tenets has been called unstructured, shared, informal, functional, empowering, participative management, consultative supervision, and joint consultation. Thus, the humanist view is much more consistent with what we have come to know as interdisciplinary leadership.

Despite the tension between these two models, most organizational literature focuses on both a technical and a human aspect. However, the human aspect of management is usually directed toward increased job satisfaction for the purpose of decreasing turnover and increasing production. And, despite the fact that structural and behaviorist models are each viewed as useful, the machine–structural model of organizations has been paramount during much of the 20th century.[5]

Models and Metaphors for Interdisciplinary Leadership

Leadership in IHCTs in the early days (1940–1975) was highly influenced by the field of group dynamics.[6] That influence was both positive and negative. Although it allowed time for tending to team process issues (e.g., encouraging every member to speak up and be heard), it did not allow enough time to establish dynamic structures that would encourage efficiency of team operation.

Development of IHCTs in the late 20th century has probably been more influenced by organizational theory and by the structural models and metaphors that have been most prominent in organizational theory. Katz and Kahn stated "that every act of influence on a matter of organizational relevance is in some degree an act of leadership" (pp. 527–528).[7] However they referred to the leadership function as directed by the formal leader. In fact, it is very difficult for organizations to give up the concept of one formal leader. And although this concept should be synergistic with informal or interdisciplinary leadership, organizations tend to ignore the informal in favor of support for formal leaders.

Although most IHCTs exist as part of larger organizations, they are not necessarily synchronous with them. If one asks health care professionals why they chose health care as a field, most will admit that it was because they wanted to help people, solve difficult health care problems, or to be in a prestigious field. They probably would not say that it was because they wanted to lead a team. The desire to lead is uttered more often by those who chose management for a profession. In management circles, interdisciplinary team leadership is usually not thought of at all or is considered a management phenomenon. In fact, it might be difficult for managers to share the leadership function with those who are not managers because legitimate authority in bureaucracies is only accepted through formal hierarchical structures. Recognition of informal leadership would contradict the basic purpose for which managers were trained.[8] This is a primary reason why interdisciplinary leadership has not been widely accepted.

Given the organizational focus on hierarchical structures and formal leadership, it is interesting to speculate what models of organization are used by those who are involved with IHCTs. One study reviewed the proceedings from the Interdisciplinary Health Care Team Conferences (1976–1985) to see if the authors advocated that teams and their leaders take on particular strategies for dealing with conflict.[9] The author categorized the papers using the four organizational frames proposed by Bolman and Deal,[10] that is, *structural* (achieve goals), *human resource* (serve human needs), *political* (use coalitions with different values), and *symbolic* (see organizational events as important for what they represent). The author found 21 of 180 articles referring to conflict. The papers advocated the human resources frame (16 out of 21 or 76%), the structural frame (4 out of 21 or 19%), the political frame (3 out of 21 or 14%), and the symbolic frame (3 out of 21 or 14%). More than one frame was advocated (6 out of 21 or 28%). The structural and political frames (to be used alone) were each advocated only once. The symbolic frame was never advocated alone and was always coupled with the human resource frame. The author speculated that the recommendation for use of the human resources frame might reflect the historical basis of IHCT (i.e., small group and group dynamics theory).

At a workshop for health care and health administration professionals, the trainer introduced Bolman and Deal's four frames by asking the participants (N = 31) which frame was primarily used by their hospital directorship and which was used by their immediate team. The responders were health care providers and administrators. Fifty-two percent thought that the structural frame was the primary management strategy used by the hospital and their immediate team. Thirty-nine percent thought that the political frame was the primary strategy used in their hospital, and 32% thought that human resource strategy was the primary strategy used in their team. The remaining participants were uncertain which strategies either the hospital or their team was using.[11]

These case studies are centered on the leadership function of addressing conflict. In reflecting on these case studies, the concern is the discordance between how health care workers think they behave, their perceptions of how they think their organizations behave, and the perceptions of those who write about IHCTs. Espousing only one or two models is not conducive to rapid change. Having access to many models of IHCT and leadership is useful for developing IHCTs that will survive within our changing times.

A third case study[12] revealed that interdisciplinary leadership is far down the list when health professionals think of IHCTs. However, there is evidence that health care professionals adopt many models and metaphors about leadership and teams. These metaphors may be different from those carried by professionals who are not in health care. Health care professionals who were members of IHCTs were asked to list the metaphors that came to their minds when they thought of health care teams. They generated metaphors that were grouped into fifteen themes. The most commonly cited theme was *chaos/conflict* (e.g., "never-ending battle, ram treatment down people's throats, dumping ground"). *Dynamic organism* was the second most commonly cited category (e.g., "plant, anthill, geese flying south)." The category of *leadership* (e.g., "collection of egos looking to Billy Martin for leadership, mountain-large base with stacked leadership and physician at top, eight-horse chariot—who's in charge and where are we going") was sixth in order of citations. All but 2 of the 10 metaphors listed in the leadership category were negative. Of those that were positive, only "soccer-balance of power and importance," reflected interdisciplinary leadership. The machine metaphor (e.g., "well-oiled machine, engine being overhauled by high school shop class, large machine with integrated functional parts"), which would fit with the structural models, was eighth in order of citations. The large diversity in metaphors cited speaks to the complexity and diversity of interdisciplinary health care practice. It also highlights the needs of health professionals for training in interdisciplinary leadership.

Leadership Theories

Although management is not the same as leadership, many individuals interchange these two concepts. The exercise of leadership by managers is characterized by the ability to reward and punish and also by the power of legitimacy.[13] Managers and administrators are designated as formal leaders. However, leadership that is exercised by those who are not formal leaders is more nebulous. Health care providers who are not formal leaders also have access to many powers of leadership including rewards (nonmonetary), punishments (usually covert), and legitimacy (knowledge or expertise). Some group researchers define nonmanagerial or informal leadership as an outcome of leadership.[14] Schön acknowledged that the role of leader can and does exist without the burdens of management and managers are not necessarily leaders. He treated leadership and management as one and suggested that anyone can perform the symbolic, inspirational, educational, and normative leadership roles that he classified as the art forms of management.[15]

If returning to the case presented in chapter 1, we find the nurse and the social worker ready to defend the need for a team to the clinic administrator who wants them to stop their weekly team meetings. The clinic physician, who was designated by the clinic as the team's formal leader, does not plan to take any action to counter the administrator's decision. He wants to accept the decision of the administrator and get on with patient care. In fact, the case does not state who is the formal leader of the clinic team. Perhaps the team has no formal leader. More likely, it is considered to be either the administrator or the physician. Perhaps the nurse and social worker should ignore the unspoken rules and assume a leadership role in this situation. It might be the only way to save the team in the clinic. Or, they might lose their jobs.

Because leadership as it is applied to health care teams emanates from the organizational literature on leadership, it is important to understand a little about organizational leadership theories. At least six categories of leadership theories have gained popularity during the past 100 years. Three of these categories constitute the earlier theories of leadership and focus mainly on "the" leader.

Early leadership theories. The early leadership theories focus on the person in the leadership role. *Trait theories,*[16] a group of early theories, propose that leaders have certain characteristics that can be measured, and like intelligence, are probably inherited. *Behavioral style theories*[17] propose that there are simple linkages between leader style and effectiveness and also that there is a taxonomy of leadership behavior. *Contingency theories*[18] combine the style and trait theories with situations in the environment that require specific approaches to leadership.

Later leadership theories. The later leadership theories focus on the culture of an organization and are characterized by *exchange theories*[19] where leader emergence depends on the possession of certain traits and on group tasks and norms for skills and values that the group finds rewarding. Anyone who exhibits competence in the group's tasks and conformity to the group's norms can emerge as a leader.[20] *Cognitive theories* include attribution theory,[21] which implies that it is knowledge of outcome that determines our imparting qualities to the leader, rather than the conventional view that it is our experience of leadership that determines outcome.[22] Cognitive models might involve scripts that are played out by organizational members[23] and person schemas where workers automatically assess traits of leaders by matching their characteristics or behavior with personal perceptions of what leaders should be like.[24] *Transformational theories* focus on establishing a goal or vision, the concept of change, and the involvement of followers in that change. Transformational leaders empower followers to act.[25] Other authors contend that in all of the cultural theories, leadership interrelates with the context from which it arises.[26]

It is clear that the later group of theories is more consistent with the type of leadership that is most useful on IHCTs. However, organizations seem to be reluctant to accept and support interdisciplinary leadership. Health care organizations, despite the high levels of educated staff, are no exception. In fact, despite the large number of publication on teams during the 1990s, organizations appear to be returning to earlier theories where leadership is focused on a leader. Leadership as an interdisciplinary phenomenon is still in its infancy.

Hollander, who noted that multiple leader roles could co-exist in groups, set the stage for informal leadership in groups.[27] Others viewed leadership as both a property of a group and a process of human communication[28] and concluded that leadership is neither the person in a formally established position nor any one person performing in the role of leader. Jago also defined the process of leadership as " the use of non-coercive influence to direct and coordinate the activities of the members of an organized group toward the accomplishment of group objectives. As a property, leadership is the set of qualities or characteristics attributed to those who are perceived to successfully employ such influence" (p. 315). This definition fits IHCTs because it does not restrict the leader to one who is formally appointed by the team, and yet it allows for addressing complexity and ambiguity. Also, leadership is seen as a dynamic process where leaders and followers exchange roles.

ESSENTIAL ELEMENTS OF INTERDISCIPLINARY LEADERSHIP

Rather than viewing interdisciplinary leadership as qualities in one person, it might be more appropriate to think of it as a system (see Figure 6.1) in which the behavior of all team members plays a role. Interdisciplinary leadership involves at least six elements (i.e., environment, situation, leader(s), team members (followers or peers), power, and communication). Communication is the constant in each of the elements. Both leaders and followers must be aware of the environment and the situations that the team must confront because they likely will need to switch roles depending on the envi-

Figure 6.1
Essential Elements of Interdisciplinary Leadership

Environment
(social structure, rules, history, politics team culture, physical setting, organization of work, structure of communication, team phase, member phase, etc.)

Leaders: Formal & Informal
(legitimacy, competence, motivations, personality characteristics, definition of the situation, knowledge of communicating, <u>power</u>)

← Accept ↔

→ Reject ←

Team Members: Followers/Peers
(expectations, competencies, personality characteristics, definition of the situation, motivations, knowledge of communicating, <u>power</u>)

Situation
(task, resources, mix of members, high stress/low stress, chosen methods of communication, etc.)

ronment, the situation, or both. Like interdisciplinary teams, the variables that comprise interdisciplinary leadership are complex and changing. The effectiveness of the leadership in any given situation will depend on the team's ability to see readily what variables need to be in place.

Environment

The team environment refers to everything (internal and external) that creates the backdrop for the team (e.g., social structure, rules, physical setting, organization of work, structures for communication, history, team culture, politics of the organization, phase of member development, and phase of team development). Social structure, organization of work, and structures for communication fit together to create the framework that helps decide what kind(s) of formal leader(s) are needed for the team. However, that decision can be tempered by the politics of the larger organization.

It is common for the administrators of a health care organization to appoint formal team leaders who are not able to support the needs of a team. It is also common for teams to organize in ways that do not support the leaders they appoint. For example, if you set up a monthly meeting with the administrative representative for the health system and the leaders of the team at a time when the formal leader of the team cannot attend it will create problems. You will get less done, you will have to double check on facts, and it will be less efficient. Although this sounds like an obvious problem, it is a frequent occurrence in IHCTs. In some cases, the physician is established as a formal team leader but is not involved in key administrative discussions with representatives of the health care system. Conversely, in cases like nursing home teams, the physician "leader" may not be involved in team discussions of clinical issues. In such cases, it is very difficult for the physician to represent the needs of the team to the larger organization, without defined structures and procedures for ascertaining the team's needs.

If some team members socialize outside the work setting, the team's culture may partially be formed without the awareness of other team members. The culture also may change with long-term or part-time team members being unaware of that change. The team needs to review regularly its culture and identify the changes as they occur.

A Changing Team Culture

In one situation an IHCT had formed with many young members and they began socializing once a week after work. As increased patient loads contracted their formal meeting time, some team business was conducted during the social hour. Gradually, the makeup of the team changed, as did its culture. Team members were slightly older with young families and some of them were unable to come to the social hour after work. The ratio of females to males increased and the few males on the team no longer came to socialize. Some team business was still conducted during the social hour, leaving members in both the old and new cultures wondering how rules had changed without them being aware of it.

The rules to which the team ascribes can be stated or unstated, made by the organization, the team, or both, and be rigid or flexible. Usually, it is not the rules that are inflexible; instead, it is the unquestioned way they are interpreted and accepted that makes them rigid. When team members interpret rules as guides to help them accomplish their mission, they realize that the rules need periodic re-evaluation, especially if the majority of current team members did not invent them.

Environmental factors such as structures for communication are extremely important and teams should review them and make their rules for using them explicit. This is particularly important as newer technologies for communication emerge. If the organization initiates a team but does not allow for structures and resources to support that team, the team will likely not perform as well as it should and will probably not survive. Organizations that do not want teams but somehow feel compelled to initiate them will frequently not assign resources to support them. If an organization sets up a "virtual team" (where members do not work from the same location) without allocating computer networks, cell phones, computer hardware, and processes for communication the team is set to fail.

Who is Responsible?

A group of professionals who worked together in a clinic called themselves a team, but had never met as a team because the clinic in which they worked had no place that was convenient and available for them to meet. The team blamed the organization. The organization didn't understand the problem.

The ways that the team environment influences leadership are limitless and should play a prime role in reviewing leadership on the team. Most of these environmental factors are malleable. However, they need to be recognized for changes to occur. Both team and organization have a responsibility to recognize forces in the environment that will be detrimental to the team.

Situation

The situation is another major variable for interdisciplinary leadership and refers to the task(s) at hand that require the team's attention. Situations that call for leadership have qualities of simplicity, complexity, normality and abnormality, straightforwardness and ambiguity, and high and low stress. The qualities of the situation should dictate which team member(s) lead and which follow. A situation might have little complexity, low ambiguity, and low stress and have too many members attempting leadership of the situation. In that case, members will be stepping on each other's toes and getting in each other's way. Another situation might be extremely complex with high ambiguity and high stress and attract one or two team members who are not trained to take on the work for which the task calls. If the environment is such that structures have been put in place for such a circumstance and the team members have been trained on an approach, they will know the protocol and know which leader to call on if the need arises.

Leaders (Formal and Informal)

Interdisciplinary leadership encompasses the complexity of the tasks that are before the team and the immediate and long-term resources that should be applied to those tasks. Each team situation that calls for leadership will involve leaders (formal, informal, or both) and team members (followers or peers).

Leading involves communication (ability to give and receive information) that is necessary for the team's work. Formal leaders are given a designated title by the organization or the team and are the types of leaders most often referred to in the organizational literature. Informal leaders can be defined as anyone who moves the work of the team forward. Team members can be formal, or informal leaders or nonleaders if they refuse to assume any leadership. Schön was one of the few organizational theorists to acknowledge that the role of leader can and does exist without the burdens of management and that managers are not necessarily leaders.[29] This brings us to a realization that members of health care teams frequently have, which is that their formal leader is not the person they are following. Health care organizations do not always appoint the most appropriate team member as a formal leader. Such appointments may be based on hierarchy of discipline and do not give sufficient consideration to the appointed leader's knowledge of leadership tasks or the time the leader can devote to such a role. Some IHCTs might be better off with several formal or informal leaders, preferably from different disciplines. It is also important that formal leaders are assigned to the team for sufficient amounts of time to perform their assigned leadership roles.

Followers (Peers)

It has been said that leaders manage meanings.[30] In this regard, team leaders interpret team events and the climate in which the events take place.

However, there can be no leaders without individuals who are willing to follow. Followers provide a context or background that invites a leader to lead. Otherwise, the leader will be seen as ineffective and will not succeed. Leadership involves considerable trust as followers accept some form of symbolic power from the leader. Because trust is such a major issue in IHCTs the accomplishment of leadership tasks is much more important than having one charismatic leader.

Some theorists view participation as the influence that comes from someone being active in decision making.[31] Expressing that influence is what followers do. There are few books written about followers, although followers are as much a part of leadership as leaders. Followers are those who are not actively assuming leadership roles, and yet have the role of accepting or rejecting leadership. All members of the team are followers at some points in time and thus all need to know how to follow. Like leading, following involves communication as the ability to give and receive information. Followers are continually assessing whether those who are leading are performing the necessary tasks of leaders; whether they as followers are adhering to the team's mission; and whether there is a gap in leadership that they have the skills to fill. The following situation speaks to the responsibility of followers in interdisciplinary leadership.

Where is the Leader?

A middle-aged female physician worked on a hospital team as well as a nursing home team and as she traveled between the institutions she was sometimes late for meetings. Although there were issues to be dealt with that did not involve the physician, the team would never start without her even when she was a half hour late. When questioned as to why they did not start the meeting without the physician, one nurse said that the team had agreed that the physician would be the meeting leader.

Power

Leaders and followers alike need to feel a sense of power and to understand their ability to contribute to the team's development and maintenance. Although there are many power sources available to team members, some sources of power have a greater potential to add value and strength to the team. Evidence suggests that leadership is related to social power because observers confer it and because the functions of leadership as a social influence process are shared throughout a group.[32] Other researchers see power in organizations as shared and deriving from activities rather than individuals.[33] Thus, the power in organizations is not static because it stems from the context of the situation and situations are constantly changing. This

fluid notion of power is similar to that of influence, defined as getting results through social interaction.[34] Social influence can also be defined as
leadership.

A study of a geriatrics team found that commitment, professional knowledge of geriatrics and/or team, energy, and dedication to improving geriatrics and/or team, were the major sources of power in a developed IHCT.[35]
Those members who had commitment to both appeared to have more power
within the team. Additional sources of power included tenure with the team
and organizational skills (i.e., the ability to organize to solve a problem).
Personal attributes like charisma appeared to be important power sources in
the early phase of a team's development. However, as the team grew, these
personal attributes became much less important. In a subsequent study,
Drinka found that the ability and willingness to teach and learn were additional sources of power for interdisciplinary leadership.[36] Thus, members
who enter a developed IHCT having knowledge, commitment, and personal
and professional values consistent with the needs of the patients to be
served will likely assume power for leadership on the team. They should
also assimilate into the team more quickly than members who have knowledge and values that are inconsistent with the patient's needs.

Charismatic leaders have a natural ability to determine the social milieu
of a situation and to shape that milieu to fit their needs. However, charismatic leaders may not play a large role in developed IHCTs. It is likely that
the more substantial power sources like commitment, knowledge, and the
ability to teach and learn will be more powerful for demonstrating leadership, at least on developed IHCTs.

THE INTERDISCIPLINARY LEADERSHIP SYSTEM IN ACTION

Tasks

If interdisciplinary leadership is really a system of interactions, it is probably not accurate to think of leadership roles. It is more accurate to think of
tasks of leadership. Rather than one role of "leader," an IHCT has multiple
leadership tasks and a multitude of opportunities to assume such tasks.
Some of the tasks of interdisciplinary leadership are seen in Table 6.1. A
member might perform many if not all of these tasks at certain times. Some
team members might perform few of these tasks. It is unlikely that a member would be able to perform all of these tasks all of the time. In general,
members of health care teams appear willing to perform certain leadership
tasks and to ignore others. Teaching health care providers how to perform

the tasks of interdisciplinary leadership should make them more willing to assume them.

In times of high stress for the team, members will likely perform the leadership tasks that are most related to their primary area of training. The leadership task that health professionals feel most comfortable with is that of "expert" in their field. Some might also feel comfortable with the tasks of "finisher, supporter, diplomat, ambassador, organizer or mover, and conformer or follower." Other leadership tasks such as process-analyzer, facilitator, challenger, and reviewer are tasks that health professionals were not necessarily trained to do, especially not across disciplinary boundaries. Yet these latter tasks are critical for the survival of interdisciplinary teams. Unfortunately, they are usually not viewed as part of professional practice, which is the reason they are the first to be ignored when a team is under stress. Some health care disciplines like social work, psychology, and psychiatry receive more training in these latter areas. However, even members from these disciplines might choose not to assume these tasks when the team is under high stress.

Matching Leader to Type of Problem

When is it appropriate for team members to fill in or to cover for other members and when is it not appropriate or dangerous to do so? To answer this question, one must take into account the different levels of professionals and paraprofessionals who might constitute the team; the amount of time each has to devote to the team; and how much and what kind of training they have had in working on interdisciplinary teams.

IHCTs have tight staffing patterns and may be constructed and staffed with part- and full-time members. In many cases, the physician is assumed to be the team leader even though he or she may be with the team the least amount of time of any other member. In this case, the appropriate assumption of leadership can be a problem.

It is important that team members know when to assume leadership and when to accept leadership from others. It is helpful to think of leadership as a way to address team problems. Problems can range from simple to complex and from common to uncommon (see Table 6.2). A simple common problem is one that occurs frequently. It might have more than one solution. However, the solutions are not ambiguous. An example of such a problem is deciding who will perform the leadership tasks at a patient care conference. Any team member can take on leadership and with proper training can perform one or more of the leadership tasks required for a successful conference. However, the team should have rules of which the team approves.

Table 6.1
Interdisciplinary Health Care Teams: Leadership Tasks

Organizer/Mover	Finisher	Expert
initiate team development identify team tasks identify strengths/weaknesses call meetings provide structure review team needs identify appropriate patients	impose time constraints focus on outputs (patients treated, goals achieved) seek progress show high commitment to task manage projects	have special expertise offer professional viewpoint identify interdisciplinary patient problems use expertise of other disciplines understand patient needs know team's expertise and limits
Ambassador build external relationships promote awareness of the team's work build bridges show concern for external team environment	**Diplomat** build understanding between members negotiate mediate facilitate decision making	**Supporter** build team morale put team members at ease ensure job satisfaction help patient work with team
Judge/Evaluator listen critically evaluate clinical process evaluate clinical outcomes help team reflect promote appropriate treatment act logically seek truth	**Process analyzer** identify team problems analyze team problems consult with team members offer observations offer potential solutions to team problems	**Facilitator** identify member conflicts help team members find ways to resolve conflicts help implement solutions

Creator	Innovator	Challenger
generate new ideas visualize new programs/projects visualize new alliances	discover resources identify opportunities transform ideas to strategy propose new methods	offer skepticism look in new ways question accepted order
Reviewer observe review team performance promote review of process give feedback mirror team's actions	**Quality Controller** check output alignment act as conscience regarding team goals inspire higher standards assure team reviews outcomes	**Conformer/Follower** seek agreement fill gaps in teamwork cooperate help relationships avoid challenges maintain continuity
Guard protect team from too much output protect team from too much input	**Teacher** help new members learn the norms and values of the team teach shared leadership skills to other members recognize members' leadership potential teach others when to seek specialty advice	**Learner** raise questions to enhance understanding across disciplines or areas raise questions regarding need for interdisciplinary input

Table 6.2
Leadership Responsibility for Different Types of Team Problems

	Simple	Complex
Common	A. Anyone can solve problem. Need rules for response to keep informal leaders from wearing out. Informal/Formal leader	C. Anyone alerts team to problem. Team designates leader and establishes practice standards Formal/ Informal leader
Uncommon	B. Anyone can alert team or solve problem. No rules; even new members are expected to take responsibility. Informal/Formal leader	D. Anyone alerts team to problem. Formal leader may want to lead or designate a leader. Formal/Informal leader

This will help distribute the tasks and keep the informal leaders from wearing out.

Any member should be able to alert the team or, with appropriate skills, solve an uncommon problem that is simple. This might involve a social worker reviewing a patient's medications or monitoring blood pressure on a home visit, or a nurse securing a ride to a clinic visit for a patient who missed his ride due to a bladder accident.

When problems are complex, any team member can take responsibility for alerting the team to the problem. However, if the problem is common, the team should designate a leader and usually establish some kind of practice guidelines so the team can try out mechanisms for solving the problem and evaluating feedback from the results. An example of a common complex problem is arriving at a format for writing interdisciplinary treatment plans. Interdisciplinary treatment plans do not focus on patient problems that are discipline specific. Instead, they see the patient as a whole individual with subsets of interrelated problems and interrelated solutions. Agreeing on a format for writing interdisciplinary problems is a complex task that requires a strong and knowledgeable leader. Having a defined format for such a common problem will increase the efficiency of the team.

When the complex problem is also uncommon, a formal leader may want to take the lead or to designate a team member as leader. Expecting a primary care clinic to absorb another clinic's geriatric population would be an example of an uncommon complex problem. A formal leader is helpful in such situations because that individual has more legitimacy with the administrative side of the organization.

Why Interdisciplinary Leadership Is Difficult

The training of health care professionals involves training in autonomous function. Leadership is focused on exhibiting skills in one professional area. Health care professionals are trained to think critically about their profession's segment of a complex problem. This is the way that most schools of health professions have been structured. Perhaps this is because this makes it easier for educators in those schools to assure that "the core body of knowledge" for their discipline is maintained. Interdisciplinary education is complicated and somewhat messy. Educational institutions are not structured to encourage cross-departmental teaching because it involves a potential loss of resources. Also, cross-departmental evaluation often involves a perceived loss of control.

The training of other health care providers is primarily technical (e.g., nursing assistants; licensed practical nurses; associate degree nurses; diet technicians; and activity, occupational, and physical therapy assistant). These individuals receive anywhere from 6 weeks to 2 years of training. Because of the technical nature of their training and the fact that they have to learn so many methodologies in such a short time, they learn to accomplish the routine procedures they are expected to perform on a daily basis. In other words, they learn to deal with simple common problems. Clinicians with more training will learn to deal not only with common simple problems, but also with "their part" of a common complex problem. They will not define a complex problem as complex because that would suggest they might have to deal with other disciplines to solve it. They will also see solutions as certain because to imagine the ambiguity would threaten their identity as a practitioner in a specific field. Instead, they are taught to see a portion of a complex problem as their problem, in effect making a complex problem simple so they can address it. There is no time to learn the type of interdisciplinary thought processes that must go into framing and solving uncommon complex problems, especially problems that are also ambiguous. There is no time to learn about the complex decision making that can create a true resolution to such an issue.

The next step is critical for understanding why interdisciplinary leadership is difficult to assume and to develop. When health care workers encounter crises as they do on a daily level, it leads to stress. As health care professionals mature, they may learn what other professions are about and what to expect from different levels of workers in those professions. They might learn to work with many different disciplines on many levels. However, this situation changes when they become stressed. Stresses for health professionals do not just come from patients; they also come from other things in their environment (e.g., conflicts with other workers, family problems, excess of work, not enough direction, changing health care regulations, etc). When the environment for health care workers is very stressful, they revert to working the way they were trained to work because that is what is most comfortable for them. They tend to lose sight of the need to work with members of other disciplines or even with other levels of their own discipline. They retreat into an autonomous mode of operation.

These comments are not meant to fault the thinking of paraprofessionals. They are intended merely to point out that, because of the training that these practitioners receive, they are limited in the scope of their practice. The problem emanates from the payment structures that are allowed in some health care situations, the making of regulations, and the clinical translation of those regulations. Focusing primarily on financial issues, health care institutions often hire the least skilled worker that is mandated to perform a job. The industry divides up health care into tasks that need to be performed rather than the health that needs to be tuned up, regulated, or restored to an individual.

ASSUMING INTERDISCIPLINARY LEADERSHIP:
EVIDENCE FOR WHY

Despite the fact that most health care professionals receive training in limited parochial leadership, there is evidence that some health care professionals can and do learn to assume interdisciplinary leadership. There is little evidence to show what conditions lead a health professional to assume this type of leadership. Drinka conducted a case study of leadership on a well-established IHCT.[37] This section addresses some of the results of that study. All of the quotations from providers are from that study.

It is helpful to review the essential elements of interdisciplinary leadership shown in Figure 6.1. In Drinka's study, the leadership *environment* on the team that was studied was a culture of valuing ideas, and the team atmosphere was one of teaching and learning. Study participants repeatedly mentioned this culture of valuing. Participants also noted that the *situation* had to be one in which they felt secure enough to assume leadership. Followers watched for models and mentors within the team. They admitted learning from them and developing a readiness for when they felt safe enough to assume leadership. Members who took on leadership often had prior experience as leader of a team. Mostly, they would take on leadership because they felt secure in doing so. None of this is surprising, except that interdisciplinary leadership appears to be a set of skills that is separate from other professional skills that members had learned. It was also different from other leadership skills that most had learned.

The merging of a team's expectations for a member to take on leadership and that team member's readiness for assuming leadership are separate but related forces that affect the leadership practices on the team. A member's state of readiness may not match the state of the team's readiness for that member to assume a leadership task. Some members appear ready to assume leadership on joining the team. Others (even well-seasoned clinicians) might feel they are not ready and hold back for months, if not years. Some members might be ready for leadership in areas such as clinical, but not evaluation or process counseling. The team's expectations of a member may prompt some *reluctant leaders* to take on a task for which they do not feel ready. Other members who do not feel ready may stand firm in rejecting an invitation to assume a leadership role.

Prior Experience or Training

Prior experience or training may be a factor in why some health professionals appear willing to assume interdisciplinary leadership, even when they are new to an established team. It appears to be part of the cognitive map that they have for themselves. A member's readiness for assuming interdisciplinary leadership tasks in a clinical area was most often expressed as a feeling that their experience had prepared them to be a leader in their field. This related to readily assuming difficult clinical roles on the team.

Interdisciplinary Leadership Related to Prior Experience and Training

From childhood on, I had always been told that I was capable and I had the expectation that I can always do what I set my mind to. I've never viewed myself as a star. I wasn't a straight A student. I wasn't scholarship material but I always was told that I was capable. So certain expectations were set out for me and I always had the feeling that I could achieve. (Nurse)

I think it is partly because I knew what I was getting into when I got here—unlike some other fellows [physicians]. Because I had done the elective and had spent a month on home care and knew that it was a team approach. And I knew a little bit about what the dynamics were. And so I was very comfortable with the approach." (Internist)

I think I had a pretty good background. Coming from the university for 10 years and floating through all of the services there doing some teaming over there. Yes, I was ready and I think I knew enough medicine to feel comfortable going into the homes and I certainly have learned a lot of medicine from the docs in particular. I had done acute care, intensive care, and the burn unit so sick people don't bother me. Frail people don't bother me. (Physical Therapist)

Natural Leaders

The concept of having *natural leaders* on health care teams appears to be alive and well. When health care professionals encounter someone who they perceive to be a natural leader they automatically have expectations that the person will assume some leadership tasks on the team. An administrative assistant remembered observing the team and choosing people who she thought would be natural leaders in certain areas. She also felt that other team members did the same thing. One team member had an interesting concept about team leaders. He felt that one could learn to provide leadership on a team but that one had to be a *natural leader* in order to lead when the team was having difficulties.

Interdisciplinary Leadership Related to Natural Leaders

And others saw it in that individual and it sort of evolves because, that person, it's apparent that they are a leader and then it just evolved and that person took it on and others encouraged it. (Administrative Assistant)

I took on leadership because I think that's my nature. I need to be able to express that. That time (when I was on the team) I was expressing that through my work. (Pharmacist)

With my friends they always naturally looked to me as somebody who has good advice who has some wisdom and that I am able to problem solve. So I think it is something that I have always done. I don't think it is something that I had to learn to do. I think it is something where you learn about different people and different personalities and learn how you can work with them and have a common goal and be able to make change. (Nurse)

Until that social worker came on board I think there wasn't a sense of leadership and I think that it was easy for the support staff to see that this new member was the person to deal with because it just seemed like it was a natural leadership role for that person. (Administrative assistant)

When the team works well, having inherent leadership qualities is less important. Then those non-natural leaders really blossom because they are able to take and run with ideas. I think that during those down times those who actually did the leading would be those who were the natural leaders, who had tough hides, and who tended not to care in the long run that someone thought it was a bad idea but would take and go with it anyway against the odds. I think that even in those circumstances, even though that person might be influential and might have a good idea, because of the nature of the team things got done very slowly if at all. (Pharmacist)

Reluctant Leaders

Although teams might have expectations that certain members should assume leadership tasks, those *chosen* members might not be ready to assume the leadership tasks that others expect of them. Sometimes, chosen members will take on the tasks despite feeling unready. Other times they won't. Some teams might be more tolerant of a member's refusal to assume leadership tasks. Other teams might not ask again even if the member feels ready at a later time. Some team members might never feel ready to take on interdisciplinary leadership. Some team members' views of leadership were more likely related to their discipline-specific role on the team and not to interdisciplinary leadership.

Comments from Reluctant Leaders

If somebody expects you to do something you just do it whether you like it or not. You were brought up that way too. You don't bitch you just do it and then you do the stuff you like to do later. (Physician who assumed a leadership role without feeling ready)

I got involved to do what I thought was a better job for myself in relation to the patient, to do more of what was expected of me and to fulfill my role better. I just simply didn't have time to worry about the team as a functioning team. I only had time
to worry about my relationship to the patient and my relationship to the team as
far as the role that I was supposed to do. And that generally took more than my job
time. (Physical Therapist who refused to take on a leadership role that was expected)

Now You See Them, Now You Don't

Some members might become involved in assuming leadership on the
team and then, for personal or professional reasons, withdraw to a less intense
level of involvement. This may be temporary (e.g., when a member returns to
school for extra training or goes on maternity leave). For some members an
initial withdrawal from leadership tasks may be the beginning of a permanent
withdrawal process from the team (e.g., a member is mandated to increase
time spent elsewhere, or a member decides to take another job). Although the
team might tolerate periodic withdrawal by a member with special expertise,
it might result in that member not being viewed as an interdisciplinary leader
by some team members. The withdrawal from leadership may be particularly
difficult for some as they will be perceived as less powerful during the time of
their absence and subsequently on their return to the team.

Thoughts on Being a Sometime Leader

The social workers were very good at teaching me boundaries at saying no. I used
to think give me everything. I can do it. But I learned that people will not think less
of you just because you say no, I'm at my level I can't do it. That was a big thing I
learned on the team. I remember the feeling of control and reduction of stress I felt
when I was given a golden opportunity to participate in this big thing and it was my
choice to at this time say no. And before that I would have felt I had to do it. (Nurse)

Leaving the team left a void. (Pharmacist)

I missed the team so much, that professional interaction and the quality of specific
team members (Physical Therapist)

I have to be able to retreat and to do what I want to do when I need to do it. And if I
am too directly involved in some activities then retreat becomes difficult because I
feel I bear a larger part of the responsibility. I don't mind being responsible for certain things but I have to limit that exposure because it risks then that I do other activities less well. (Physician)

Additional clues as to why team members may or may not assume leadership might be found in some of the metaphorical themes generated in the
study by Drinka and Miller.[38] "Resentment of the physician as leader (ab-

sentee landlord)" might prompt a "natural leader" to fill in the leadership gap, especially if they are a long-term team member. Looking at leaders as "a bunch of unfriendly quarterbacks" might keep a potential leader from assuming leadership tasks and risk being identified with that group. A "stalemate" metaphor might also keep potential leaders from assuming leadership in a team culture where everyone is waiting for someone else to make the first move.

It is important that IHCTs not close the door on any member's potential for leadership. For some individuals it might take more time, more training, or simply more professional maturity to be willing to assume leadership. Some team members may never be ready. It would be helpful to make the expectation for interdisciplinary leadership explicit in the primary training that professionals receive.

ASSUMING INTERDISCIPLINARY LEADERSHIP: EVIDENCE FOR WHEN AND HOW

Strong Feelings

The when and how members assume leadership tasks are tied together and difficult to separate. Also, a range of variables regulates when and how members assume leadership. Themes from the study by Drinka[39] included strong feelings about an idea or a situation; expectations by self and others; and development of a commitment or a common trust between the team and the member who was targeted for leadership. The major triggers for involvement in a leadership role included a sense of enthusiasm or excitement about an idea or issue or a sense of frustration or anger about a situation. Combined with the excitement, there was considerable evidence that team members recognized the added work responsibility accompanying the assumption of leadership as a trade-off for self-defined job satisfaction. Associated factors included length of experience in clinical practice, availability of formal leadership roles in the team, and percentage of time the member was assigned to the team. Some members chose to get involved early in their tenure, whereas others spent several years observing the team to assess the nature of their future leadership role or a leadership role for another member of the team.

Excitement as a Stimulus for Assuming Interdisciplinary Leadership

I took on a leadership role because I felt very strongly about some of the issues that were coming up and so I felt like if I wanted to make changes that I thought were important that I should get involved. (Physician)

We did it because it was exciting. It was a challenge and there was fun about the team being a bastard outside of two big bureaucracies and to this day we carry the stigma and resentment of some people because of that attitude that we manifested and the way in which we operated but we also achieved. And nothing is perfect so I guess I don't know that we have to be. (Nurse)

It was just so exciting. And then we wanted to let everyone else know about it because it was this great thing and we were doing this great stuff. (Social Worker)

It feels good if you can make an impact and change things to make them better for the patient as well as staff satisfaction. (Nurse)

I was learning something new and I love to learn. I have memories of some very high energy discussions in the hall with people, things that we were excited about and thought we ought to be able to investigate, things that we could do to grow. So I guess just in terms of generating ideas I think that it wasn't so much my role in doing that but that I had a need to do that. That was part of what made it stimulating to stand around with team members and talk about what we could do if we had the resources. (Psychiatrist)

I did have an interest in being involved in something that was innovative. That was enough motivation there to be involved in that. (Occupational Therapist)

That's a buzz. When you get a roll going with this stuff it is just a kick. (Occupational Therapist)

I find it gratifying to work alongside other people on projects having them appreciate ideas that I come up with and being able to work with them on those ideas. (Psychiatrist)

In almost all instances there was a payback to me personally in that being able to motivate this group of people. There was an incredible amount of support aside from actually joining in and helping to get the job done it was sort of the recognition, of the accomplishments and the completion of the task. That you could really feel good about it without having to worry if it was in your area of specialty or not. Both of those made it incredibly easy. Also, it was an incredible learning process. (Pharmacist)

Frustration as a Stimulus for Assuming Interdisciplinary Leadership

I changed the policy because it was something that I felt so strongly was a waste of time. (Physician)

I was motivated because it was a problem that was dissatisfying either to myself or to others as well. (Administrative Assistant)

I was angry. I mean I felt that the system was basically designed so the patient could always call the same audiologist, social worker, or whatever but I felt the patients were not getting good medical care. It was so haphazard in how it was being performed. I felt the physicians were always being usurped, basically by the team members to the detriment of good patient care. (Physician)

Because I had some expertise in that area or an interest in it. I got involved with the treatment plans because the ones we did initially I considered just busy work. You wrote on them and you never touched them again until two months when you had to write on a separate sheet of paper, re-write all your goals and all of your objectives. I thought that was a waste of time that I didn't have. (Nurse)

Just the fact that you are a doctor you are legally and morally responsible for the patient. If it is directly associated with a patient you have to facilitate it and if you don't you are a mess. (Physician)

I do have an idea of what is correct almost all of the time. Even if things aren't black and white there is a better way for most things, to initiate therapy or treat a patient. So you get involved to get it done the best way, and maybe prevent a lot of the big time problems. (Pharmacist)

If we did something a little different we could either anticipate what was going to happen to the patient or provide them more or better service. (Physician)

I get involved because if you don't get involved when you see a change coming or you see the need for change you don't have any say in what happens. Things change around you and you are totally out of control. (Social Worker)

Some of the things that would come up at times were sort of disruptive, and it felt like they were undermining things that were there and were okay. But there was a lot of it that I could agree with when it resonated with my own sense of feeling repressed. That was sort of a prompt for a more productive discussion for how we could change things. And so I think some of the less idealistic, I have to make my job better, kind of complaining was another factor. (Psychiatrist)

I can remember lots of times the hallway discussions we would have were bitch sessions and I think that kind of complaining sometimes also generated new ideas and impetus for change. (Psychiatrist)

Some tasks of leadership that are appropriate during one phase of a team's development are not necessarily those that will work at another phase of a team's development. Also, because team members may be at different phases of development, a particular task of leadership may be more relevant for some than for others. There is no way that one designated team leader could be expected to perform all of the tasks of interdisciplinary leadership that an IHCT needs to grow and maintain itself.

TEAM MEMBERS' PERCEPTIONS OF LEADERS

Each team member can usually identify the formal team leaders. Team members seem less certain about who the informal leaders are in a particular situation. Health care providers who are seen as informal leaders by their teammates may be reluctant to view themselves as leaders. Drinka[40] studied the development of leadership and the perceptions of team members in an IHCT that had evolved over a period of fifteen years, with no assigned internal leaders and with little direct formal leadership. This study focused on whether or not formal and informal leadership developed within the team, how leaders developed, and what made team members assume leadership roles.

Thirty-four team members were asked to identify the members of the team who were leaders during each time period that they (the interviewees) were members of the team. Over a span of 8 years, there were nine separate time periods representing periods of stable team membership. Data on a member's perception of self and others' perception of a member are compared in Table 6.3. This table lists data by professional discipline, gender, percent of the time an individual rated self as leader out of the number of times possible, percent an individual was rated by other members as a leader of the number of times possible, the direction and percentage of the difference, years on team, percentage of time on the team or whether that percentage varied, and whether a member had a formal administrative role on the team.

Self-Perceptions of Being a Team Leader

There was variety in the team members who perceived themselves as leaders of this IHCT. Team tenure appeared to be a major factor in establishing a self-perception of interdisciplinary leadership. Members with longer tenure generally had stronger perceptions of themselves as leaders than those with shorter tenure. However, neither discipline nor gender of the member seemed to be a factor in whether a member perceived him or herself as a leader or in his or her perception of the consistency of leadership over the years he or she was a member of this team. It was no surprise that those who had formal leadership roles were more apt to perceive themselves as leaders than those who did not.

Team Members Perceptions of Others as Team Leaders

Data from Table 6.3 on members' perception of others as team leaders revealed that members differed in terms of who and how many members in a given time period they perceived as leaders. Members did not necessarily view the same members as leaders in all time periods that they were on the team. Some team members did not list other members as leaders during time periods when those members demonstrated physical or emotional absences from the team. It is clear that team tenure did play a role in that longer tenure tended to increase the chance of a member being perceived as a leader. Also, formal leadership role seemed to be associated with being perceived by others as a leader. However, a formal leadership role did not guarantee that others would perceive a member as a team leader, especially if those being rated were transient members of the team. No member of this team was rated as a leader 100% of the time. This indicates that even the highest rated leaders were not always matching some members' perceptions of leadership. The members who at times did not perceive the team's needs for leadership as met, even by the highest rated leaders, tended to be those who were themselves perceived by others as leaders.

As the qualitative data in this study were compared to the quantitative data it became clear that several other factors assured that members would be perceived as leaders. Members who were seen as either extremely competent clinicians or as extremely creative problem solvers were seen consistently as leaders. Finally, when members appropriately assumed the leadership task of process analyzer, it assured them of being perceived by others as powerful leaders on this team whether or not they had a formal leadership role.

Team members who were not perceived by others as team leaders tended to be newer members (less than 3 years) of the team. The one factor that almost guaranteed that members would not be perceived as leaders was whether they had been forced to join the team or felt like they had no other choice. There were times when administrators would assign someone in their department—often someone who was seen as a misfit in his or her department—to the team. If joining the team was something that a clinician did not want to do, it made it difficult for that person to assimilate into the team and almost impossible for that individual to assume any interdisciplinary leadership tasks.

Large Differences in Self-Perception and Others' Perceptions of Team Leaders

Perceptions of leaders varied by team member. Each member appeared to have a perception of who the leaders were for any given time period of

Table 6.3
Selected Characteristics of All Team Members During a 9-Year Period

Profession/ Discipline	Gender	A-Self perception (%)	B-Others perception (%)	Difference A-B (%)	Years on team	Time devoted to team (%)	Formal leadership role
R N	F	100	98	+2	>3	100	Y
M D	F	100	91	+9	>3	V	Y
S W	F	100	91	+9	>3	V	Y
PSY	M	100	89	+11	=3	V	N
S W	F	100	85	+15	>3	100	Y
M D	F	0	75	-75	<3	V	Y
O T	F	0	75	-75	<3	50	N
P T	F	83	74	+09	>3	25	N
A A	F	0	74	-74	>3	100	Y
M D	M	100	66	+44	>3	V	Y
R N	F	71	63	+08	>3	100	Y
S W	F	—	63	—	<3	V	Y
S W	M	0	58	-58	<3	100	N
R N	F	75	57	+18	>3	V	Y
P H	M	100	55	+45	>3	V	N
S W	F	—	55	—	>3	100	Y
M D	M	—	55	—	<3	V	N
R N	F	—	53	—	<3	50	Y
R N	F	—	53	—	<3	50	Y
R N	F	0	53	-53	>3	V	Y
P T	F	0	50	-50	<3	V	N
M D	M	100	47	+53	>3	V	Y

128

PT	F	0	44	44	<3	50	N
PH	F	40	44	-04	>3	40	N
MD	M	0	43	-43	=3	>	N
RN	M	0	42	-42	<3	100	Y
MD	F	0	42	-42	<3	>	N
PSY	M	100	40	+60	=3	>	N
OT	F	0	39	-39	<3	50	N
OT	F	—	36	—	>3	>	Y
MD	M	—	36	—	<3	>	Y
RN	F	0	36	-36	<3	50	N
MD	F	0	35	-35	<3	>	N
MD	M	100	32	+68	<3	>	Y
RN	F	50	31	+19	<3	>	N
MD	M	—	29	—	<3	>	N
RD	F	—	26	—	<3	50	N
RD	F	—	25	—	<3	50	N
MD	F	0	22	-22	<3	>	N
OT	M	—	21	—	<3	50	N
PSY	F	—	21	—	<3	>	N
OT	F	0	20	-20	<3	50	N
PT	F	0	19	-19	>3	>	N
MD	M	0	16	-16	<3	>	N
MD	F	50	14	+36	<3	>	N
MD	F	—	14	—	<3	>	N
PH	M	0	10	-10	<3	40	N
RD	F	—	07	—	<3	50	N
MD	M	—	06	—	<3	>	N

team membership. These attributions or cognitive schemas pertained to both the member's perception of self as leader and the member's perception of other team members as leaders. Every member of the team had a discrepancy between the percentage of time they perceived self as leader and the percentage of time others perceived them as leader. However, some members had a large discrepancy (> 19%) between how they rated themselves and how others rated them as leader. There was greater than 19% discrepancy for 21 (8 out of 11 males and 13 out of 23 females) of the 34 members who performed this exercise (see Table 6.4). Gender appeared to be a variable in either greatly overestimating (male) or greatly underestimating (female) one's self-perception of leadership. The trait of physician was also associated with greatly overestimating one's self as leader on the team. And male physicians seemed to be the most prone to believing that they were exhibiting team leadership when in fact they were not, or at least it was not being recognized as such by the team. Another study described those who overestimate their authority as naive group members and noted that those individuals usually characterized themselves as natural leaders.[41]

Administrators often expect physicians to assume the role of formal leader. Despite this expectation of leadership, physicians often have limited leadership training and heavy time commitments. While physicians expect to assume leadership on IHCTs, they might not be the most appropriate health professional to assume a role like team coordinator. Also, the nature of a patient's perceived problems might dictate the assumption of the leadership role of care coordinator by team members who are not physicians. The high status of the profession of medicine establishes the strength of this double bind.

The female leaders in Drinka's case study[42] appeared to be unsure of their informal leadership potential and the impact of their informal leadership on the team. Because this is a case study, it is not possible to extrapolate to female members of other health care teams. However, it is possible that females tend to greatly underestimate their potential as leaders of health care teams. Also, little team longevity and low percent time on the team cannot be underestimated as factors in creating faulty perceptions of leadership.

Table 6.4
Members with Greater Than 19% Discrepancy
Between Self-Perception and Others' Perception of Leader

	Overestimate	Underestimate
Males	5	3
Females	1	12

N=21 of 11 males and 23 females who performed the exercise

We need to think of mechanisms that will close this gap between the perceptions and realities of leadership, especially if we are talking about health professionals job sharing, working on multiple teams, or making virtual teams work. IHCTs are complex social systems that exist within other complex social systems. As such, we should expect that the leadership of IHCTs would be a complex phenomenon. Rather than thinking that we can identify certain traits of leaders, it may be more helpful to identify situations in which leadership should play a role and members are expected to assume leadership tasks. The concept of singular leader should be abandoned because no one leader can provide all the leadership in any complex situation. Instead, we might think of opportunities for leadership in a leadership system.

ADDITIONAL LEADERSHIP RESPONSIBILITIES

Patients and Team

Although the patient's role in the team has been addressed in articles on teamwork, this is a controversial area that has not been well defined. Like team members, patients must at times assume the tasks of leader and follower. Although patients are not core members of the team, they are at the core of the team's decisions and the team's work. The capacities of patients to participate in their care differ markedly. The very nature of being a patient means that one needs someone with more knowledge about certain areas of health care. This need puts patients at a perceived power disadvantage and perhaps it is why they are often reluctant leaders.

Patient as Reluctant Leader and Unwilling Follower

Marty is a relatively healthy well-educated young male who is depressed and has been seeing his primary care doctor for treatment. "I just got a call from Dr. B.'s nurse about my blood level and it was very high. However, she had remembered that I had asked if time of day mattered (the time the blood was drawn). So she began asking around (Dr. B. is out of town) and no one on the team seemed to know anything. Apparently there are supposed to be at least 12 hours between taking the drug and the blood draw. At best there was a 10–hour difference. I can't imagine that it will make a big difference since the reading was so high, but, I will go back and let them draw again tomorrow morning. The high level might explain the tremors I have been having in my arms and hands. I asked another physician who I know and she said that this medication has a long half-life (time it takes the level of medicine to drop in half) and that 2 hours wouldn't make any difference in the blood level. I am not sure why they waited to do a blood level, probably a cost-saving measure that enters into their evaluation at the end of the year. First I was too low, then I got pushed to an appropriate level and was doing fine, so instead of leaving the dosage alone Dr. B. increased it hoping that would move things along more quickly. I called him a few days after I started taking the higher dose to tell him that I didn't feel well but he just said that he would wait to get a level when I returned for my regular appointment. Now I am at too high a level and am having all kinds of problems. I am thinking of finding another physician, but I have been going to Dr. B for so long and I don't know who might be good. I would like to decrease the dose, but I don't want to do it without his permission. Next week when Dr. B. is back I am going to encourage him to refer me to a psychiatrist."

What began as a relatively simple and common case had the potential to become complex. To avoid that probability it required communication and a team effort between the nurse, internist, a psychiatrist, and Marty. That did not happen soon enough and Marty was hospitalized.

This case reflects the ambiguity that many patients feel when they know something is wrong but they don't know how to engage the team in a way that will assure them the best care. It is not clear who has the responsibility to teach patients how to participate in their care and how to most effectively interact with the team. Currently, the popular press attempts to teach patients how to interact with their physician. However, this is a complex topic and little is done to address the patient's relationship to the team.

Administrators and the Team

The team and the organization that houses the team have an obligation to see that the patient knows the team's members, what they are trained to do, how they work together to provide care, and what their options are if they feel they are not getting the care they need. The patient has an obligation to keep track of treatment effects and to be honest and open with the team. The team has the daunting task of learning what kind of care the patient and family want and integrating that knowledge with their expertise at providing care. This is a dynamic process that requires good communication between the patient and team systems.

Administrators have an obligation to be interdisciplinary leaders as they provide vision and resources for the team to perform its work. They are also expected to be followers by observing and evaluating the team's work and attending to areas where they can help the team to succeed. They must listen to the needs of the patients through the collective eyes of the team and translate that knowledge into the ever-changing world of health care financing.

SUMMARY

This chapter began with the definition of interdisciplinary leadership as moving the work of the team forward. As we end the chapter we would like to present a revised definition.

Interdisciplinary Leadership Is:

- Moving the work of the team forward
- Directing the practice of health care toward the needs of the patient and the viability of the system
- Using uncommon sense in common situations

NOTES

1. Bolman, L. G., & Deal, T. E. (1984). *Modern approaches to understanding and managing organizations.* San Francisco: Jossey-Bass; Morgan, G. (1997). *Images of organization* (2nd ed.), Thousand Oaks, CA: Sage.

2. Morgan, *Images of organization.*

3. Bass, B. M. (1990). *Bass and Stogdill's handbook of leadership: Theory, research and managerial applications* (3rd ed.). New York: The Free Press.

4. Bennis, W. G. (1965). Theory and method in applying behavioral science to planned organizational change. *Journal of Applied Behavioral Science, 1,* 337–360.

5. Morgan, *Images of organization.*

6. Baldwin, D. C. (1996). Some historical notes on interdisciplinary and interprofessional education and practice in health care in the USA. *Journal of Interprofessional Care, 10,* 173–187.

7. Katz, D., & Kahn, R. L. (1978). *The social psychology of organizations* (2nd ed.). New York: Wiley.

8. Pfeffer, J. (1981). *Power in organizations.* Marshfield, MA: Pitman.

9. Drinka, T.J.K. (1987). Interdisciplinary health team and organizational development literature An analysis of approaches to conflict recognition, resolution, and management. In M. L. Brunner & R. M. Casto (Eds.), *Interdisciplinary health team care: Proceedings of the eighth annual conference* (pp. 74–84). Columbus: School of Allied Medical Professions and Commission on Interprofessional Education and Practice, The Ohio State University.

10. Bolman & Deal, *Modern approaches.*

11. Drinka, T.J.K. (1986). Unpublished data.

12. Drinka, T.J.K., & Miller, T. F. (1996). The health care team as metaphor: A preliminary study. *Journal of Allied Health, 25*(3), 247–261.

13. Katz & Kahn, *The social psychology of organizations.*

14. Cartwright, D., & Zander, A. (1968). *Group dynamics: Research and method* (3rd ed.). New York: Harper & Row; Vroom, V. H., & Jago, A. G. (1988). *The new leadership: Managing participation in organizations.* Englewood Cliffs, NJ: Prentice-Hall.

15. Schön, D. A. (1984). Leadership as reflection in action. In T. J. Sergiovanni & J. E. Corbally (Eds.), *Leadership and organizational culture: New perspectives on administrative theory and practice* (pp. 36–63). Chicago: University of Illinois Press.

16. Stogdill, R. M. (1948). Personal factors associated with leadership: A survey of the literature. *Journal of Psychology*, *25*, 35–71; Terman, L. M. (1904). A preliminary study of the psychology and pedagogy of leadership. *Journal of Genetic Psychology*, *11*, 413–451.

17. Lewin, K. R., Lippitt, R., & White, R. K. (1939). Patterns of aggressive behavior in experimentally created social climates. *Journal of Social Psychology*, *10*, 271–299; Stogdill, R. M., & Coons, A. E. (Eds.). (1957). *Leader behavior: Its description and measurement*. Columbus: Bureau of Business Research, The Ohio State University.

18. Bales, R. F., & Slater, P. (1955). Role differentiation in small social groups. In T. Parsons, R. F. Bales, & E. A. Shils (Eds.), *Family, socialization and interaction process* (pp. 259–306). Glencoe, IL: The Free Press; Hersey, P., & Blanchard, K. (1982). *Management of organizational behavior: Utilizing human resources* (4th ed.). Englewood Cliffs, NJ: Prentice-Hall; Hollander, E. P. (1964). *Leaders, groups and influence*. New York: Oxford University Press; House, R. J. (1971). A path-goal theory of leader effectiveness. *Administrative Science Quarterly*, *16*, 321–338.

19. Graen, G., Novak, M. A., & Sommerkamp, P. (1982). The effects of leader–member exchange and job design on productivity and satisfaction: Testing a dual attachment model. *Organizational Behavior and Human Performance*, *30*, 109–131; Hollander, E. P. (1979). Leadership and social exchange processes. In K. J. Gergen, M. S. Greenberg, & R. H. Willis (Eds.), *Social exchange: Advances in theory and research* (pp. 103–118). New York: Winston-Wiley.

20. Bass, B. M. (1990). *Bass and Stogdill's handbook of leadership: Theory, research and managerial applications* (3rd ed.). New York: The Free Press; Smith, P. B., & Peterson, M. F. (1988). *Leadership, organizations, and culture*. London: Sage.

21. Calder, B. J. (1977). An attribution theory of leadership. In B. M. Staw & G. R. Salancik (Eds.), *New directions in organizational behavior* (pp.179–204). Chicago: St. Clair Press.

22. Smith, P. B., & Peterson, M. F. (1988). *Leadership, organizations, and culture*. London: Sage.

23. Argyris, C. (1982). *Reasoning, learning, and action: Individual and organizational*. San Francisco: Jossey-Bass; Argyris, C., Putnam, R., & Smith, D. M. (1987). *Action science*. San Francisco: Jossey-Bass.

24. Foti, R. J., Fraser, S. L., & Lord, R. G. (1982). Effects of leadership labels and prototypes on perceptions of political leaders. *Journal of Applied Psychology*, *67*, 326–333.

25. Bass, B. M., Waldman, D. A., Avolio, B. J., & Bebb, M. (1987). Transformational leadership and the falling dominoes effect. *Group and Organization Studies*, *12*, 73–87; Bennis, W., & Nanus, B. (1985). *Leaders: The strategies for taking charge*. New York: Harper & Row; Burns, J. M. (1978). *Leadership*. New York: Harper & Row.

26. Smith, P. B., & Peterson, M. F. (1988). *Leadership, organizations, and culture*. London: Sage.

27. Hollander, E. P. (1961). Some effects of perceived status on responses to innovative behavior. *Journal of Abnormal and Social Psychology, 63*, 247–250.

28. Fisher, B. A. (1986). Leadership: When does the difference make a difference? In R. A. Hirakawa & M. S. Poole (Eds.), *Communication and group decision-making* (pp.197–215). Beverly Hills: Sage; Jago, A. G. (1982). Perspectives in theory and research. *Management Science, 28*, 315–336.

29. Schön, Leadership as reflection in action.

30. Morgan, *Images of organization*.

31. Vroom, V. H., & Jago, A. G. (1988). *The new leadership: Managing participation in organizations*. Englewood Cliffs, NJ: Prentice-Hall.

32. Lombardo, M. M. (1978). *Looking at leadership: Some neglected issues* (Tech. Rep. No. 6). Greensboro, NC: Center for Creative Leadership.

33. Salancik, G. J., & Pfeffer, J. (1977). Who gets power—and how they hold on to it: A strategic contingency model of power. *Organizational Dynamics, 5*, 3–21.

34. Parsons, T. (1960). *Structure and process in modern societies*. New York: The Free Press.

35. Drinka, T., & Ray, R. O. (1986). An investigation of power in an interdisciplinary health care team. *Gerontology & Geriatrics Education, 6*(3), 43–53.

36. Drinka, T.J.K. (1991). A case study of leadership on a long term interdisciplinary health care team (Doctoral dissertation, University of Wisconsin-Madison, 1990). *Dissertation Abstracts International, 51:11*, 3599A.

37. Ibid.

38. Drinka, T.J.K., & Miller, T. F. (1996). The health care team as metaphor: A preliminary study. *Journal of Allied Health, 25*(3), 247–261.

39. Drinka, A case study of leadership.

40. Ibid.

41. Beckhouse, L. S., Tanur, J., Weiler, J., & Weinstein, E. (1975). And some men have leadership thrust upon them. *Journal of Personality and Social Psychology, 31*, 557–566.

42. Drinka, A case study of leadership.

7

Conflict and Problem Solving as Indicators of Team Function

CONFLICT ON INTERDISCIPLINARY HEALTH CARE TEAMS

When health care providers from multiple professions and different levels of training are assembled in a team and expected to function, it can be anticipated that there would be conflict. Unfortunately, just mentioning the word *conflict* elicits fear in many health care providers. Perhaps it is the discomfort that comes from thinking that conflict will impede the progress of work that is often burdensome and that conflict will place us further behind. Or, perhaps it is that health care providers see themselves as helpers to people in need. If conflict is viewed as primarily negative, it seems out of place in a helping situation. Although they might see themselves at odds with a few patients, providers do not see themselves as being in conflict with them. There are a few articles written about interprofessional conflict among health care providers from different disciplines. There is little written about conflict within teams, or about conflict between team members and patients or about conflict between IHCTs and administrators. Despite this, conflict does exist in all of these venues and that conflict comes in many varieties. The conflict that relates to team members might be open, but more often it is veiled behind the cloak of the life-saving activities in which we busy ourselves.

In the past, most interprofessional literature was concerned with reducing conflict.[1] Relatively few articles in the interdisciplinary health care team literature have addressed conflict and even fewer have addressed it as a positive force.[2] And yet, conflict management might be the process factor that is most necessary for both innovation and survival of IHCTs.[3]

Much has been written in the general literature about using conflict as an impetus for positive change. In fact, conflict can also be seen as an essential part of team function and maintenance, because it is inextricably tied to innovation, evaluation, and effective problem solving. Methods for constructively confronting conflict allow team members to move a team beyond its basic group development tasks and to promote frequent re-evaluation of its established norms, goals, procedures, and outcomes. Skills in conflict management and integrative problem solving are necessary for team members who assume the leadership role of teaching teamwork. And, evidence of constructive confrontation is an indicator of an IHCT's readiness to model teamwork.[4]

Types of Team Conflict

Intrapersonal. In discussing conflict, it is helpful to determine who is feeling the effects of the conflict. When you feel the burning in the pit of your stomach that so often results from conflict, it is tempting to think that the whole world is at war. However, intrapersonal conflict may only exist within one individual. In fact, you might be the only one who is feeling negative effects from an experience as a team member. While "The Meeting" incident described here may reflect bad behavior on the part of the team, this appears to be an intrapersonal conflict.

The Meeting

Jane was fairly new to the team. However, she had worked on other IHCTs and felt comfortable expressing her viewpoint in the team's meetings. A team member objected strongly to something that Jane said in a team meeting. In unison, the whole team said, "No, we don't want that." Jane kept quiet for the rest of the meeting. She felt terrible and was sure that the team did not like her. Jane's stomach began to hurt and she was beginning to doubt why she took the job. Several days later, Jane approached one of the team members to ask why everyone at the meeting was so vehemently opposed to her idea. The team member told Jane that they had tried that idea within the past year and found it to be dangerous to patients. The team member assured Jane that no one was upset and that they realized she wasn't involved in the problems the idea had created.

In the case of "The Meeting," it is possible that the team could harbor ill feelings about Jane for bringing up an issue about which they had negative memories. Also, intrapersonal conflict can quickly affect the team. If Jane were to act differently toward the team because of what she experienced in the meeting, this could turn into another kind of conflict. If a nurse comes, sleep-deprived, to work after a major argument with his spouse, the nurse's mood will likely affect his interactions with other team members and, in subtle ways, with patients. We like to think of ourselves as professionals who leave our personal problems at the door. However, we are only human. Because conflicts escalate so quickly they are seldom of one type. Many interpersonal and intrateam conflicts start as intrapersonal conflicts.

Interpersonal. Interpersonal conflict occurs between two individuals. In relation to IHCTs, this type of conflict could be between two team members. It could also be between a team member and a health care practitioner who is either part of the same health care system or part of another health care system. Another type of interpersonal conflict could be between a team member and a patient or member of the patient's personal support system. Because of the speed with which health care providers often work, it is sometimes difficult to recognize and check interpersonal conflicts at an early stage. When interpersonal conflicts are not recognized they can rapidly escalate to intrateam or interteam conflict.

A Real Pain

Sue had been referred for a magnetic resonance imaging (MRI) scan of her spine. Having had previous MRIs, Sue remembered that they were loud. She kept telling herself that she would remember to ask for a pillow under her knees and earplugs for her ears. In the interaction with the technician, Sue remembered the pillow, but forgot to ask for earplugs. After the first set of pictures, the technician asked Sue how she was doing. Sue told her that she was very uncomfortable because of the loud noise and asked if she could have earplugs. The technician told Sue that she would have to start over if she brought Sue out. After the procedure was completed the technician suggested that if Sue was bothered by noise she should have asked for earplugs before the procedure. Sue asked the technician why earplugs couldn't be placed on the table for the patient to decide. The technician said that was not feasible because in the last several months Sue was the only person who had asked for earplugs.

It is important for health care providers to see complaints from patients as information for problem solving. Disgruntled patients are likely to seek out new health care providers, write letters to administrators, and contact attorneys.

Intrateam. Intrateam conflict is conflict that may start out between two members and grow to involve either part of the team or the entire team. When team members begin taking sides against another group of team members intrateam conflict exists. The entire team might also be pitted against one of its members, viewing that member as the scapegoat.

As explored in chapter 4, intrateam conflicts are often about professional values where members of one profession view a situation differently from those of another profession. When intrateam conflicts form along disciplinary lines it is a sure sign that the team or some of its members are in, or have reverted to, an early norming phase or even back to the forming phase of development. Intrateam conflict can occur over differences in values between two subcultures of the team. In addition to professions, those subcultures might be grouped by values that spring from any similar quality (e.g., age, gender, having to miss time at work because of problems with child care, or distractions because of ill parents).

Intrateam conflicts can also generate creative dialogue between team members who have achieved the confronting or performing phases. The nature and openness of the conflict are indicators of whether the conflict is healthy or unhealthy. The openness of the problem may also be contingent on how the conflict is defined by different members of the team.

Creative Approach to Intrateam Conflict

A physician who worked on an IHCT that delivered home care was disenchanted with the format of the interdisciplinary care plan. She openly complained to the team about how awkward it was to write in the current format and also that it was not easy to follow the patient's progress. The team challenged the physician to change the care plan. The physician took up the offer and asked for team members to work with her in developing a new prototype for the plan. Team members also suggested other members who they thought could contribute to restructuring the plan. The volunteers formed a subcommittee with the physician and developed a draft of a new format that they brought to the team for comments. The new format was adopted and became one of the most successful innovations of this team's history.

Unproductive Approach to Intrateam Conflict

A physician who worked as part of an IHCT clinic team did not like the way the clinic functioned. He was constantly complaining that it was inefficient and not well organized. He decided that he would invite the physicians who worked in the clinic to meet him in a bar after hours. He wanted to get the physicians' input regarding a plan that he had developed for changing the clinic operation. After the physicians who met in the bar had approved the new clinic plan, the physician who started this process presented his plan to the clinic coordinator who was a social worker. The social worker, although skeptical of the new plan, suggested that the recommendations be presented to the entire team for input. Because the other physicians in the clinic had already agreed to the plan, when it was formally presented to the team its adoption was assured. The revised plan did not help clinic efficiency and made the nonphysician members very unhappy. Within several months the plan began to fall apart and within a year all traces of it were gone from the clinic.

Interteam. Interteam conflicts are true system conflicts. They can occur within one system between an IHCT and another part of the system or between two different teams in separate systems. In an era of limited funding by health insurers and limited support by some agencies, it is common for patients to move between health care agencies or between clinics within the same agency. This can cause conflict between health providers who don't normally work together as they are forced to communicate. This is conflict that cannot be ignored.

The Case of George

George, an elderly man with many chronic health problems, lived alone and had been treated by a home care team for several years. George's beloved dog died about the same time that George developed throat cancer. One day, the nurse made a home visit and found George wandering aimlessly in his backyard. She quickly realized that he was hypoxic and suspected that the tumor in his throat was closing off his trachea. George was quickly rushed to the hospital where it was the policy for the inpatient team to "take over" a patient's care. Aside from a transfer note or discussion, the home care staff was discouraged from visiting a patient until discharge was imminent. Several days after admission the home care staff received word that George was agitated, was constantly pulling out his tracheostomy, and in a hypoxic state was ripping off his clothes. The inpatient nurses were upset because they were unable to communicate with him. George's living will stated that he wanted everything possible done for him. A speech pathologist was called in and tried to teach George how to communicate with a communication device. The physician came in and told George that he would not live if he did not keep his breathing tube in. The inpatient social worker called George's friends and minister. George refused to communicate with anyone and continued to pull out his tracheostomy tube and rip off his clothes. On a hunch, the home care social worker stopped by George's room and asked him if he wanted to go home. George shook his head in the affirmative. The home care social worker promised George that if he would keep in his breathing tube for 2 days she would try to take him home for a visit. This time George remained intubated. The next few days were hectic as the home care staff negotiated the trip home. The hospital team was against the visit and members were certain that George would not return to the hospital. On the third day after George left in his tracheostomy, three members of the home care team (nurse, physical therapist, and social worker) signed George out of the hospital against medical advice and took him home where his neighbors and minister met him. The minister held a prayer meeting and George's friends took him to each room of his home so he could say goodbye. When the home care staff returned 3 hours later George was ready to return to the hospital. Two days later George died peacefully in his sleep. The hospital team continued to express anger at the home care staff.

Handing off cases to other teams, organizations, or family members is a major source of interteam conflict. If the two teams do not jointly define the problem there will likely be conflict. In the case of George, the inpatient team wanted to give the patient the best care possible and they defined the care as reducing hypoxia. The home care team was defining best care as increasing George's quality of life in his last days. If both teams had defined the problem together there likely would have been much less interteam conflict and George might not have suffered as much as he did.

Sources of Team Conflict

We have discussed four types of team conflict. However, there are many more sources of team conflict. Each of the components in the IHCT model that was presented in chapter 2 (see Table 2.1) is a potential source of team conflict.

Components that directly influence practice. Unique characteristics of each member, coupled with the strengths and knowledge each member has in his or her profession, can be strong sources for team conflict. For example, a nurse who grew up in a family whose members avoided confrontation at all costs would be influenced by that background. If that nurse was not very secure in his or her profession, the nurse would be even more likely to avoid conflict. On the other hand, being a risk-taker can be a source of conflict on a team where the other members are very conservative. A recently trained professional can be a source of conflict on an IHCT that has little turnover and where the members have not learned how to mentor or learn from a new member.

Intrateam components. Internal structure and process components can all become sources for conflict. Structural issues like physical placement of offices can be a major source of conflict when team members are not near each other and have not established structures for informal interaction and communication. Internal process components like problem setting can be a source of team conflict when patient problems are identified as discipline-specific and charted according to actions by individual disciplines. If there are no structures or processes set up for conflict management or for teaching new members, or if the structures and processes established for these components are ineffective, conflict will ensue.

Organizational components. Any of the components that relate to the internal organization or to external organizations that affect the team can be a source for team conflict. If a health care organization establishes IHCTs and continues its discipline-specific methods of evaluation rather than team-specific methods, that will be a source of conflict for the teams. If state and national policies for reimbursement do not support the use of IHCTs with patients whose needs are complex and ambivalent, there will be conflict. Health care providers will be stressed and the patients will be upset for not receiving care that addresses them as whole persons.

Components for team maintenance. An IHCT must have a way of collectively identifying its accomplishments and needs. If an IHCT does not regularly present its accomplishments and needs to the larger system it will be a source of conflict. The larger system is apt to only look at the direct team costs and begin to think of the team as a liability. If the large system does not have a forum for receiving the needs of a team it will be a source of team conflict.

Not knowing what you don't know. When health care providers are sure they understand something that they don't it can be a recipe for disaster. This is a common source of team conflict, in teams that use ad hoc or formal work group methods of problem solving. It is also a major source for conflict between members of an IHCT and those who are not members—patient, family, or other teams—especially when hand-offs occur.

The Hand-off

A family practitioner, the only member of her group who had been fellowship trained in geriatrics, had recruited older patients with complex and ambiguous problems into her clinic. She had also assembled a small IHCT consisting of a nurse and social worker. For the first time in 3 years, the geriatrician decided to go out of town on vacation. She asked her physician colleagues if they felt comfortable covering for her while she was out of town for 2 weeks. The physicians laughed and one of them said, "Oh that won't be a problem, we'll expect a few calls about adjusting Digoxin doses." The geriatrician replied that they would be more likely to receive a call in the middle of the night from a distraught caregiver because her elderly mother who has Alzheimer's has been found wandering around in the snow. The physicians decided that they should further discuss the call procedures. Because the geriatrician had the physicians' attention she also told them what they could expect from the team members who were not physicians.

Professional autonomy and fear of making mistakes. There are two additional sources of team conflict that are worth mentioning because they universally apply to health care professionals. They are *professional autonomy* and *fear of making mistakes.* Both of these sources of team conflict are linked to the cultures within the health professions and the training each profession mandates to retain that culture. These aspects of training within each profession are reflected in the difficulties they experience with teamwork. The performance of an IHCT is based on admitting that different disciplines are needed to effectively treat a patient population. The team must assure a common definition of a patient's problems and open communication between the disciplines to determine type and sequence of interventions. Because a team's growth is based on its ability to evaluate itself and to correct its mistakes, members of IHCTs must be willing to trust all team members to observe the team's work and give honest feedback.

We have stated that the schools of health professions train students to function autonomously. Their leadership training does not teach interdisciplinary leadership, but rather it trains professionals to lead their professional colleagues. When health care providers must teach or give feedback to team members from other disciplines, it crosses a boundary they were not trained to cross and creates uncertainty, fear, and intrapersonal conflict.

Health care professionals are trained not to make mistakes. However, health care inherently addresses life-and-death issues for patients who are at risk from illnesses that might not be fully understood. Consequently, health care is fraught with mistakes. And, health care providers will admit to mistakes in private conversations with providers of their own kind. Some disciplines, like physicians, are taught to learn from their mistakes in venues like "tissue conferences" or "peer review." However, this learning is meant for physicians and is not meant to be interdisciplinary. And although these learning venues are common in academic settings during training, they do not necessarily carry over to nonacademic practice situations. If admitting mistakes to members of one's own profession is difficult; admitting mistakes across disciplinary boundaries is unimaginable for some professionals. In establishing an IHCT, interprofessional trust is established. This trust is the foundation for sharing mistakes across disciplinary boundaries. IHCTs must establish safe interdisciplinary venues to learn from their mistakes. The organization that houses the team must build these venues into their formulas for financing teams. Without such a mechanism, there will be little learning across disciplinary boundaries and the IHCT will not be able to grow as a team and its value of freely integrating knowledge in complex cases will be lost.

Peer Review

An IHCT initiated a process of interdisciplinary peer review. Annually, each team member was to fill out a short written evaluation on every other team member. The intent was to give constructive feedback. After the first round of evaluations, the physicians in the clinic stopped the process because they said that members from other professions did not have the knowledge to evaluate their work.

Limited time, uncertainty, and constant change. The appropriateness and quality of team decisions will be based on members' abilities to problem solve in the context of conflict. The stresses of limited time, uncertainty, and constant change couple with the team's components and past training to produce conflict. Such conflicts enhance health professionals' fear of relinquishing autonomy and admitting mistakes. Thus, it is imperative that team members feel comfortable in recognizing problems with patient care and in discussing these problems (including their mistakes) with their teammates. This requires that, early in its existence, the IHCT establish acceptable mechanisms for interdisciplinary reviews of patient care and team function. If written peer review is unacceptable, then an open forum for voicing concerns is necessary. When a mechanism for review is not jointly defined and mutually understood it will not work and will only cause more conflict for the team and regression to an earlier phase of team development.

Reactions to Team Conflict

As much as we would like to think of ourselves as rational beings, our responses to team conflict will involve some kind of emotion and that emotion will manifest itself in numerous ways, direct and indirect, verbal and non-verbal (see Table 7.1). These emotions are expressed in conjunction with the various approaches we take to managing conflict. Using different terms, researchers have outlined five approaches to conflict management—*coercing/forcing, avoiding/withdrawing, compromising/negotiating, accommodating/obliging*, and *collaborating/integrating*.[5] The chosen approach is driven by past experience, training, motivation, and habit. These five approaches can also be thought of as avenues to problem solving. To productively use any one of the five approaches requires knowledge of the power requirements, desired outcomes, and appropriateness of an approach for a given situation (see Table 7.2). A major departure from previous work is the acknowledgment that in the process of collaborating on an IHCT, power within the team is frequently not equal, but every member must have power for decision making.[6] It is at the level of integrative problem solving that the power lies with the team. An increased level of IHCT development and a greater depth of culture will allow team members to freely exercise each of the five conflict or problem-solving styles and will channel individual styles toward a collaborative approach. As an IHCT matures it should become more proficient at selecting the conflict or problem-solving approaches that are the most appropriate for a given situation.

If conflict is not addressed it tends to escalate and erode the trust and commitment of team members. When we ask health care providers to name the approaches to conflict that they think are most commonly practiced by

Table 7.1
How Team Members Express Emotions in Conflict Situations

Direct-Verbal	Indirect-Verbal
describe feelings: (consistent with the core values and ground rules that the team has set) focus only on one point blame others deny one's actions over defend a position	raise or lower voice raise unrelated points change opinion when pressured expand guilt verbally attack members over unrelated issues
Direct-Nonverbal	**Indirect-Nonverbal**
withhold relevant information exclude essential disciplines	be silent glare laugh or grunt sigh obey with rancor avoid eye contact slouch or sit erect fold or wave arms tighten facial muscles conceal emotions

health care professionals, the answer is usually collaboration and accommodation. It does not help that most conflict-style assessment instruments
allow people to think that collaboration is their preferred style of conflict
management. However, when using more sophisticated conflict management instruments like The Conflict Management Survey[7], it becomes clear
that the preferred styles of health care providers are avoiding and coercing.
Coercing and avoiding behaviors that emanate from fear of making mistakes can impede open dialogue with other providers. In fact, coercing and
avoiding are intertwined. Although many people think avoiding is passive,
it is actually an active style of conflict management. A team member cannot
coerce another member unless that person is willing to avoid or withdraw.
Also, if someone actively avoids a conflict situation long enough the
avoider becomes a coercive force.

As a way to cope with their intrapersonal and team conflicts, team members often become masters of avoidance. If health care professionals perceive that they do not have time or do not know the appropriate strategies for
confronting and resolving conflict, they will avoid it. They are more apt to
avoid it in the forming and norming phases of team development. Table 7.3
demonstrates some of the many avoidance mechanisms used by health care
providers to address conflict. The use of avoidance as a primary coping
style impairs the ability of the team to function creatively and efficiently. By
virtue of their training, health professionals feel that conflict should be
avoided. However, their habits, motivation, and past experience may
change that avoidance to coercion.

Stress and conflict trigger amazing things in IHCTs. Conflict can be used
as an impetus for the team to innovate and grow. However, if members are
continually stifled or coerced in terms of their change efforts, then team
members may try to serve their own self-interests by turning on other team
members. It is helpful to look at the types of conflicts that are occurring and
how they are being dealt with in order to understand how to make them
productive.

We all have experienced behaviors of a clerk or waitperson who is
stressed. If we see the conditions of the stress or are somehow aware of
them, it is much easier to accept a longer wait for service. However,
when the clerk or waitperson is exceptionally friendly, smiles, and says
things like, "I will be right with you" or "your order is on its way" and
nothing happens for a reasonable length of time, feelings of helpless
frustration result. It is equally frustrating when a team member uses a
cheerful style to avoid some conflict that has occurred or is occurring. In
effect, this person is denying the conflict and choosing the avoidance
style of the "sunshine club." This behavior is particularly forceful when

Table 7.2
Using Conflict to Promote Interdisciplinary Problem Solving

METHODS/STRATEGIES	POWER

Coerce-Force/
One defensive; one offensive;
  emphasize differences; judge &
  accuse
	Imbalance (real or perceived);
	  attempt to retain imbalance

Withdraw-Avoid/
One defensive; one offensive;
  emphasize differences
	Imbalance (real or perceived);
	  attempt to retain imbalance or
	  create new imbalance

Negotiate-Compromise/ Bargain; hoard information	Relatively equal; attempt to increase relative power

Accommodate-Oblige/
Share all information, clarify all
  disagreements; equalize input
	Relatively equal; attempt to further
	  equalize power

Collaborate-Integrate/
Openly present problems; use all
  power strategies; balance
  conflict & cooperation
	Universal and unequal; members
	  free to get more power; team
	  controls power for decision
	  making

CONCLUSION	USE/DON'T USE
One yields or standoff	Emergency; unpopular issue, fixed resources, need decision/ Need support or long-term relationship
One yields or standoff	Trivial issue; little power; nonrecurring problem; part of larger problem/ Serious issue; critical goals; recurring problem
Different factions agree to accept decision; all win and lose	Mutually exclusive goals of moderate importance; balanced power; focused on roles/ Early in problem; need more information
Overt agreement; covert disagreement	When wrong; need social credits; goals not critical; to promote member responsibility/ Issue important to team and relationships
Comprehensive solution & re-evaluation	Critical needs & goals; ill-defined problem; need commitment/ No time; no trust

Table 7.3
Avoidance: The Team's Favorite Conflict Management Style

1. **Patients come first.** Ignoring the concerns of a co-worker on the pretext that you need to attend to the needs of a client, all the while planning to avoid the co-worker's concerns.

2. **Strong emotions (blowing smoke).** Someone begins yelling at you regarding mistakes that were made. This takes the heat off of them because they realize that they have contributed to the mistake.

3. **Intellectualization.** If you cite authoritative sources you can usually avoid the conflict of being questioned.

4. **Rationalization.** If a person doesn't want to constructively approach a conflict, he or she can always find an excellent (and very rational) reason not to do so.

5. **Negativism.** "Yes but," "that won't work," "we've tried that" are all expressions of negativism that put people off and keep them from offering what might be important suggestions to alleviate the conflict.

6. **Procrastination.** Focusing on things that are "more important" because you really don't want to deal with the conflict: "I know I have to deal with this, but the patients come first."

7. **Humor.** Using humor to divert the focus from the problem so the problem never gets addressed.

8. **Compulsivity.** Focusing more intensely on the task to get it "perfect": "Maybe if we just keep doing this and get it right the conflict will go away."

9. **Slowdown.** Doing the task very slowly so that you don't have to face the conflict: "I'll do this, but maybe if I work slowly they will forget about it."

10. **Bringing in food.** It is difficult to address a conflict toward you if you have just engaged in such a "kindness."

11. **Positivism.** "Of course we can do that," "we do that all the time," "we already do that" are avoidance responses when used as a way to keep people from improving the process.

12. **Sunshine club.** "I don't know what you are talking about; we don't have a problem" is an especially powerful avoidance response when it involves team members who are leaders.

13. **Sick in.** A team member does not show up for a meeting or team training because they claim to be sick.

14. **Half-truths.** Addressing the less difficult parts of an issue temporarily gets the monkey off your back.

15. **E-mail.** When you are upset, using e-mail as a way of communicating with a colleague avoids directly confronting a significant conflict or issue.

16. **Beepermania.** Continually being beeped out of meetings. The beeper controls the individual and allows them to use it as an excuse for avoiding unpleasant situatons.

Table 7.3 (continued)

17. **Do what I know best.** I'll just do my own job and not make any waves. What is going on around me is none of my business even if it is affecting the team.

18. **Robert's rules of order.** Using strict rules to avoid all conflict—even when it might be constructive.

19. **Too busy—no time.** Thinking that we are so important that we cannot take the time to resolve a conflict.

20. **It would upset the patient.** Using a patient as a shield to avoid conflict.

21. **River in Egypt.** Denial is very effective in assuring yourself that a conflict really does not exist when the evidence suggests otherwise.

22. **Anything could happen.** Using vague but seemingly serious personal medical conditions keeps others from confronting you.

powerful team members engage in it. Situations like this are even more frustrating when they involve communications problems within a system in which a team is working.

Sunshine Club

A team pharmacist approached the formal leaders of an IHCT (a nurse and a physician) to suggest that there was a lot of conflict among team members because some had not been properly oriented and others resented that the newer members did not know how to work on a team. The formal leaders rejected the suggestion that the team was in conflict, saying that everything was fine and suggested that the pharmacist was a "negative" person. As more new team members became disgruntled and left the team the pharmacist went to the administrator at the next higher organizational level to repeat what he had stated to the formal team leaders. The administrator said that he had heard nothing but good news about the team's function from the two leaders and suggested that there really was no problem.

MATCHING THE TYPE OF CONFLICT TO THE PROBLEM-SOLVING RESPONSE

Conflict and the Phases of Team Development

Conflict strategies as an indicator of team function. The methods that a team uses to address or avoid conflict can be a predictor of that team's ability to function. They can also be used as an indicator of the team's current phase of development. Although conflict is present in all phases of a team's development—forming, norming, confronting, performing, and leaving—it is addressed differently in each phase.

In the forming phase, members are guarded and unsure of their purpose. Conflict cannot be readily seen because it is neither discussed nor addressed. In the forming phase, conflict can be caused by differences in members' expectations concerning why they are on the team, expectations and uncertainty about what each team member will do on the team, about fitting in, and about not embarrassing one's self or profession. These conflicts are often intrapersonal conflicts and are seldom discussed. Accommodation may be overused in this phase. Coercion may also be heavily used in the forming phase. It is easy for one member to coerce other members in this phase because they are relatively quiet as they try to find their places on the team.

In the norming phase, members begin to recognize that they do not agree on the collective goals and purposes of the team. Scapegoating is common behavior for a team that is in the norming phase of development. It is probably not unhealthy for teams to have scapegoats as long as the scapegoats do not last for more than a few days. When a member remains the team's scapegoat, it exemplifies a deeper problem and perhaps reveals a team that is stuck in this phase. By allowing oneself to remain a scapegoat, a team member might indicate that he or she is stuck in an early phase of team development even though the team might have progressed to another phase.

In the norming phase, members develop an expectation for "equal power." Team members might want to rotate leadership tasks in order to avoid conflict and maintain "equal power." In this phase, the team adopts policies as mechanisms to avoid open conflict. One team that was stuck in the norming phase imposed *Robert's Rules of Order* on itself. These were used during patient care conferences and prevented the team from addressing the difficult issues that kept it from maturing. Addressing conflict in writing keeps the source of the conflict hidden. Members might address ongoing team conflicts with written policies and procedures where negotiation will be cautiously used. Frustration would be expected to build in the advanced norming phase with an increase in defensive communication. Members might try to force ideas on other members as they struggle to retain their equal power. Other members will avoid confronting aggressive team members as a way of retaining their "equal power." As the team approaches the confronting phase, conflict will begin to erupt. This conflict may frighten some members who withdraw to the overtly more comfortable norming phase.

In the confronting phase, there may be increased conflicts over values, leadership, equality, and commitment. Again, the methods team members use to confront each other in this phase are a measure of the team's development. If some members use coercion and others counter with avoidance there will be confusion as to which members are being coercive and the result will be a reversal of members back to the norming phase. When some members realize the power of constructive confrontation and use the opportunity to engage in problem-solving behavior, interdisciplinary leaders begin to emerge. As more members assume appropriate leadership tasks, there will be a realization that member power is not equal. To use conflict to its fullest potential, all members must begin to realize their unique potential for power that enables the assumption of interdisciplinary leadership. In this phase, the members need to focus on framing interdisciplinary problems in ways that promote the assumption of power by members who have the skills to contribute to the resolution of a specific problem.

Unproductive Confrontation

A well-developed IHCT was under extreme pressure to produce—even while clinic administrators were reducing physician staff. Several years previously, one of the team members had left her position as nurse on the team to become a part-time administrator and educator to this and other teams. While the position cuts were looming, one of the physicians approached the educator and in a condescending voice said, "What do you do anyway?" The physician wanted the former nurse to return to clinical nursing to take some of the burden off the team. Rather than discussing the source of the cutbacks or whether the physician's unspoken idea made any sense, the physician devalued the educator's work and made the position of educator seem worthless. The educator was caught off guard and became defensive. Nothing productive was accomplished.

This is an example of two members of a team that was functioning somewhere between confronting and performing in its development when it was bombarded by some very unusual stresses. This unproductive confrontation accomplished nothing because the two individuals involved were both using coercion and the outcome was a stalemate. The physician and nurse could have accomplished a positive confrontation by jointly defining the interdisciplinary problem with all of its variables. They could have brought the issue to a subcommittee for the team or to a team-process meeting. In defining the problem, the nurse and physician should have focused on what the clinic was expected to accomplish (e.g., whether the clinic had the right mix of disciplines, whether the procedures for seeing patients could be streamlined to save time and still deliver quality, and what else could be done to alter team stress). The nurse and physician likely regressed to a norming phase of development and hopefully they returned to the confronting phase and were able to open this issue and turn it into a learning experience that was valuable for the team's growth. If the entire team had returned to the norming phase, nothing positive would have been accomplished and the anger would have grown.

The IHCT moves into the performing phase when there is consistent evidence of constructive confrontation among members. Individual members feel free to demonstrate their power in the process of integrating solutions to team problems. In the performing phase, members might assume advanced teaching roles and protect the rights of their fellow members to use power.[8] By establishing individual power as a norm, the team assures that a few members do not assume all of the power on the team and that every member has power for decision making. Performing can be seen when the conflicts are directed more at program development and efficiency than at individual members. Also, the differences of each team member become an appreciated addition to the team. Members have discussed differences in values and trust each other enough to view conflicts as normal. Both the ongoing team members and the entire team might continue to re-cycle through different phases as they encounter new problems.

Repeated unproductive conflict propels some team members to leave the team. The conflict might come from within the team, an individual, or the organization. Sometimes leaving is contagious and more than one team member decides to leave. A team member from such a team drew a picture at a team workshop. She depicted her team as a graveyard with names of the exiting disciplines on the gravestones. Mass emigration often results from unaddressed conflict and can propel the remaining team members into the leaving phase. An IHCT that is stuck in this phase spends most of its energy on grieving, allowing little energy for interdisciplinary problem solving.

Relating Power Currencies to Conflict and Styles of Problem Solving

In the chapter on leadership we discussed the power sources that are available to members of IHCTs. There are other kinds and uses of power that are also important in the management of team conflict. Every team member has access to and is susceptible to the use of power currencies. Power currencies are tangible and intangible attributes that are valued by people. They are things like respect, information, morality, trust, influence, enthusiasm, ambition, assertiveness, skills, well-being, orderliness, efficiency, logic, integrity, warmth, friendliness, openness, flexibility, beauty, and wealth. They can be any attribute that an individual finds attractive. In fact, these are the things that motivate people. Advertisers focus on attributes that consumers value in order to sell products. In the process of communication colleagues and teammates use *power currencies* to "get our attention." Power currencies can form the magnet that attracts one to a certain individual. We might be attracted to people because we value trustworthiness and see them as trustworthy. Health professionals in general have strong affinities for the power currencies of respect, morality, knowledge, helpfulness, and integrity.

As the fire that warms also burns, power currencies can be used in both helpful and destructive ways. In fact, the same power currency can be used with any of the conflict or problem-solving methods. For example, if a team wanted to coerce the pharmacist by using the power currency of "respect," team members could say, "We will lose all respect for you if you neglect to give the patient the pain medication that he or she needs." On the other hand, the team could also choose to use any other problem-solving style with the same power currency of respect. Using collaboration or integration they might say, "We are concerned that the patient is truly suffering; we respect your knowledge of the patient and wonder how we can discuss possibilities for more effective pain control." When health care workers overvalue a certain power currency, others might use that currency in coercive or avoidant ways to sway the workers to a specific way of thinking. Although coercive and avoidant methods of problem solving sometimes have their place, they do not lead to creative solutions for difficult problems.

Coercion in a Team Meeting

A pharmacist was upset because the team physician prescribed a particular antihypertensive drug. The pharmacist knew that the team valued knowledge and accuracy and chose a team meeting to ask, "Why was this drug prescribed when it has such terrible effects on orthostatic hypotension?" The venue of the meeting and the pharmacist's tone and words were coercive. The team physician became defensive and retorted with more coercion. If the pharmacist had approached the physician alone or with another involved team member they could have engaged in an ad hoc problem solving session and solved a problem before it got out of hand. If there were broader issues, those issues could be brought to the team.

Even if an individual does not value a particular currency but knows that others overvalue it, that person may use that currency in various ways to manipulate members to one way of thinking. Because there is often a fine line between problem solving and manipulation, the main concern is that the team's culture, in the face of conflict, promotes both freedom to problem solve and freedom to dissent.

Addressing Ongoing Maladaptive Behavior on the Team

As social human beings, we all engage in behavior that can be construed by others as manipulative and potentially maladaptive. Because we value certain power currencies we formulate our communications in a way to draw people to our viewpoint. When we are stressed, we are more likely to use coercive methods. If those with whom we communicate do not share our values or perceive that we don't share theirs, they might view our communication as manipulative. For example, if a team social worker continually refers to his or her job as advocating for patients, other team members will think that they are seen as not advocating for patients. This is why it is so important for team members to make their values explicit and teach each other what knowledge they bring to the team. Clarifying positions and perceptions will stem some of the maladaptive behavior that will inevitably strike the team.

Behavior that is maladaptive and potentially destructive to the team is part of every team's fabric. Unfortunately, maladaptive behavior that leads to conflict tends to be ignored by both health care providers and those who write about IHCTs. One of the few articles about maladaptive behaviors on an IHCT gave examples of maladaptive behaviors and discussed them as an intrateam phenomenon in terms of willing and unwilling participants as conduits, receptors, and reflectors.[9] The article also gave suggestions on how team members could recognize maladaptive behaviors and address them at the individual, dyadic, and team levels. Prior to publication, this article was rejected several times because reviewers refused to believe that maladaptive behavior is a problem on IHCTs. However, on publication numerous comments from readers indicated that these behaviors are very common indeed.

Team members, knowingly and unknowingly, can become active and passive participants in a team's system of maladaptive behavior. If a team member chooses to engage in maladaptive behavior he or she as *originator* can initiate a message that is sent to a *receptor(s)*. Receptors accept the originator's message without question because the message is consistent with what they believe or because the individual giving the messages exhibits qualities prized by the receptors. *Conduits* transfer messages to other team member receptors who may or may not be the intended target of the message. Reflectors reflect praise to the originator, as a reminder that he or she is valued. All of these keep the maladaptive system going.

Although maladaptive behavior might be associated more with certain members than others, it is also dependent on the background situation (e.g., the mix of providers in a given situation, the stress level of members, the maturity of the team, and the support and involvement of the broader organization in the team's well-being). It is helpful to look at the use of power currencies and maladaptive behavior at the team or system level where sometimes even compliments can be perceived by some as coercive.

A Web of Maladaptive Behavior

A nursing assistant who valued efficiency finished her patient care duties before all of the other nursing assistants. A supervisor complimented the nursing assistant for being so efficient and recommended her to the administrator for a special award. Another nursing assistant resented the attention given to the efficient assistant. The slower assistant as the originator appealed to the caring nature of several other assistants and, using them as receptors and conduits, mentioned that she felt the assistant who had received the award did not spend enough time with patients and really did not care for them. These words changed the viewpoints of other nursing assistants who passed along these negative comments and actively excluded the efficient nursing assistant from their breaks, lunches, and parties. They also agreed to collectively work at a slower pace. As this collective behavior intensified, some of the other nursing staff wanted to complain but were convinced by the slower assistants that the efficient assistant did not take enough time with patients and did not really care about them. Because the nursing assistants seemed united, the nurses believed them. The team members chose not to talk with the efficient assistant because they did not want to offend the other assistants. The efficient assistant became very distraught and decided to take a job in the kitchen.

USING CONFLICT TO DEVELOP AND MAINTAIN THE TEAM

Acknowledging Team Conflict

The most important step in managing conflict is to recognize it as conflict. This recognition must be an ongoing and accepted part of maintaining the team. It is not safe to assume that the formal leaders of an IHCT will be the ones to recognize and address team conflict, because to do so might be perceived by them as failure. Conflict is usually first recognized by those team members who are closest to it or most deeply affected by it. The members who are affected first might also be those who have assumed few informal leadership tasks because they are the ones who are most intensely watching and learning. Because the leadership tasks of judge, process analyzer, facilitator, challenger, and reviewer are some of the most difficult, there may be IHCTs where no one is willing or able to assume consistently these tasks. If these tasks are left unfilled, there is a high probability that a team will become embroiled in unproductive conflict and that conflict may end up destroying the team.

Conflicts can be an important source of innovation in group decision making.[10] Conflicts can either force team members to search for better solutions to underlying problems or they can lead to mediocre or undesirable solutions. Producing innovative solutions depends on encouraging and capturing creative suggestions early in their development, even if they provoke conflict. Establishing safe venues for expressing conflict is one of the most useful things that a team can do. However, establishing them can seem like a team is caught in a catch-22. In a study of a developed IHCT, a feeling of comfort with the team was one of many variables associated with assuming and teaching team leadership tasks.[11] Promoting healthy disagreement in the form of constructive confrontation is a leadership task for advanced team leaders. And yet, if members do not feel safe, they will never assume these difficult tasks. The challenge is establishing an IHCT with structure and process mechanisms in place for acknowledging conflict.

The team can teach all new members how to recognize and address conflict and how to engage in one-on-one confrontation at the interpersonal level. New team members with skills in handling conflict can be targeted to learn and quickly assume specific leadership tasks that identify conflict at the intra- and interteam levels. Meetings can be designed to allow time to address conflicts. Rules can be established that do not discourage conflict or the acknowledgment of it. Members can be trained to look for team metaphors or slogans that either encourage or discourage conflict and to make use of those that encourage constructive confrontation. For example, the slogan, "united we stand, divided we fall" might increase cohesiveness, but will not likely enhance creative efforts.

Monitoring and Managing Team Conflict

It is helpful for team members to stand back and analyze conflict situations. By doing this members may discover that they are using an approach that no longer fits the situation or maybe never did. Values, procedures, or structures can keep a team from an impasse when there is too much or too little conflict. Table 7.4 is a guide that will help team members know what interventions are needed in many types of conflict situations.

One strategy in maintaining a team is to assign a team facilitator to monitor and manage conflict. It is often most effective to choose someone as facilitator who is not a clinical member of the team. Unfortunately, not being a practicing clinician on the team excludes the facilitator from the most valued status of member. Although this makes it more difficult for the facilitator to gain legitimacy with the team, such individuals will quickly prove their worth because conflict is just around the corner. Ideally, the facilitator would be someone who is trained in interpersonal dynamics and who understands the nature of IHCTs. Such people are difficult to find and may be seen as expendable when budgets are cut. Health care organizations should think more about the cost of establishing a team and about the benefits and efficiencies of maintaining a team once it has been established.

Table 7.4
Promoting Constructive Conflict on Interdisciplinary Health Care Teams

Domains	In General	Approach for Too Much Conflict	Approach for Too Little Conflict
Values	Clarify differences and similarities between individual and team culture of teaching and learning	Focus on interdependence of team members	Emphasize importance of open questioning in a learning environment
	Increase sophistication about intrateam relations	Review dynamics and costs of escalation	Clarify costs and dynamics of avoiding
	Increase awareness of feelings and perceptions	Share perceptions and clarify issues as a team	Raise consciousness about informal leadership
Procedure	Modify within-team procedures	Increase expression of within-team cohesion	Increase expression of within-team differences
	Train team leaders to monitor team climate	Expand collaborative strategies	Teach constructive confrontation
	Monitor team behavior	Teach members skills of process analyzer	Teach members the skills of process analyzer
Structure	Encourage organizational interventions	Use organizational hierarchy	Exert pressure for better performance or new approach
	Develop regulations	Establish rules for interactions	Eliminate procedures that stifle conflict
	Create new roles for team communication	Integrate roles of subcultures	Assign leadership tasks of challenger, judge, process analyzer
	Redefine team boundaries and goals	Redesign team to emphasize task	Clarify tasks for informal leadership in patient care and team process

Establishing Team Standards or Values for Conflict

Creating rules for conflict management is extremely important and can be done early in a team's formation. A team will want to re-evaluate these rules as it matures. Teams often ignore establishing standards for conflict management by using some of the avoidance strategies already mentioned. Because conflict management is not a priority when all seems calm, the establishment of standards might not get done at all. A team might not see the value of having standards for conflict management until a major conflict paralyzes the team. Table 7.5 is a set of rules that could provide a team with ideas on what they might want in their practice standards. These rules are only suggestions. It is most useful if each team establishes its own rules and the members agree to adhere to them. The standards should be clarified for prospective team members before they agree to join the team.

Table 7.5
Rules for Health Care Teams

1. Commit to establishing a climate of questioning and open discussion.
2. Everyone has an obligation to disagree if they feel they can improve on an intervention.
3. Everyone has the obligation to give each other honest feedback (e.g., "my perception of your role on the team is . . . ; I appreciate it when you . . . ").
4. Disagree at the cognitive level (e.g., focus on tasks and on differences about how to best achieve common objectives) versus the affective level (e.g., focus on personal incompatibilities or disputes).
5. Recognize that there may be several valid approaches to a situation.
6. Each member teaches new members the mission, values, and norms of the team.
7. Team members follow through on commitments made at meetings.
8. The team establishes a plan to evaluate itself on an ongoing basis.
9. Start and end meetings on time; turn off all beepers or check them with a secretary.
10. Use meetings for issues that need to be discussed by the full team; presentations to the team are direct and to the point.
11. Separate patient care meetings from administrative team meetings.
12. Use agendas and assign someone the responsibility for each item before the meeting.
13. One person talks at a time, while the others listen and don't interrupt.
14. Create solutions that benefit as many parties as possible.
15. Assign complex issues to subgroups to bring new information back to the team.
16. Draft agenda for the next meeting at the end of each meeting.
17. Agree on an action plan before the end of the meeting. Allow enough time for this to happen.
18. On areas of conflict, continue open discussion outside the meeting only among team members.
19. Review and evaluate each meeting (e.g., have each member give one sentence about what was good and what could be improved).

SUMMARY

If a team's culture develops based on principles of individual professional culture and autonomy, the team is not interdisciplinary and will probably not see any value in interprofessional conflict. Although a team's culture is not a tangible commodity, it will be understood by the team's members and is one of the first things that a new member will notice. Establishing rules for team conflict is helpful, but it is not sufficient to assure that a team will use conflict to its advantage. An IHCT that is well functioning will, over time, develop a culture that values conflict. In fact, the value a team has for conflict will become part of that team's culture. An IHCT that is well functioning will have a culture that views conflict as an essential element for team growth and innovative problem solving.

NOTES

1. Kane, R. A. (1975). *Interprofessional teamwork* (Manpower Monograph No. 8). Syracuse, NY: Syracuse University School of Social Work.

2. Drinka, T.J.K. (1987). Interdisciplinary health team and organizational development literature: An analysis of approaches to conflict recognition, resolution, and management. In M. L. Brunner & R. M. Casto (Eds.), *Interdisciplinary health team care: Proceedings of the eighth annual conference* (pp. 74–84). Columbus: School of Allied Medical Professions and Commission on Interprofessional Education and Practice, The Ohio State University.

3. Drinka, T.J.K. (1994). Interdisciplinary geriatric teams: Approaches to conflict as indicators of potential to model teamwork. *Educational Gerontology*, *20*, 87–103.

4. Ibid.

5. Blake, R. R., & Mouton, J. S. (1964). *The managerial grid.* Houston: Gulf; Thomas, K. W. (1977). Toward multi-dimensional values in teaching: The example of conflict behaviors. *Academy of Management Review*, *12*, 484–490.

6. Drinka, Interdisciplinary geriatric teams.

7. Hall, J. (1986). *Conflict management survey.* Woodlands, TX: Teleometrics International.

8. Drinka, T.J.K. (1991). A case study of leadership on a long term interdisciplinary health care team (Doctoral dissertation, University of Wisconsin-Madison, 1990). *Dissertation Abstracts International*, *51:11*, 3599A.

9. Drinka, T.J.K., & Streim, J. E. (1994). Case studies from purgatory: Maladaptive behavior within geriatrics health care teams, *The Gerontologist*, *34*, 541–547.

10. Morgan, G. (1989). *Creative organization theory.* Newbury Park, CA: Sage.

11. Drinka, A case study of leadership.

8

Team Members as Learners and Teachers

Participating as a health care provider on an IHCT is an educational experience. Learning, as a health professions student, how to become a member of an IHCT is also an educational experience. These statements reveal at once a fundamental principle of teamwork and a thorny problem for educators and trainers who work with practicing teams or students in the health care arena.

The fundamental principle is that teamwork is an experiential learning process: learning occurs by doing something, by actually working collaboratively with other health professionals. This approach is in contrast with the didactic instructional method typically used to teach core knowledge content in health professions education—for example, a course on physiology or anatomy. On the other hand, it is consistent with the basic approach of clinical instruction, which is hands-on and "real world." Unfortunately, most clinical instruction occurs in a unidisciplinary fashion, where the student is exposed primarily to the same health profession.

The thorny problem is that currently practicing clinicians and students working on teams may have very different perceptions of whether learning is occurring, how it is happening, and the significance of that learning for themselves as individuals and for the team as a whole. Often, health care professionals seem to act as if learning stops when they graduate from their respective programs and start work as a clinican in the "real world." In the case of teamwork, they may just assume that they should be able to become part of an IHCT and have all the knowledge and skills they need to perform well in this role. Managers and administrators may contribute to this problem by creating "teams" and assigning members to them, without thinking about the significant challenges of learning to collaborate—especially when individual professionals are socialized into very narrow disciplinary roles and know relatively little about what other health professions really do.

Thus, the educational issue becomes one of revealing the true nature of interdisciplinary teamwork: that it is fundamentally an experiential learning activity; that it is based on a perspective of lifelong learning as a professional; and that it demands energy, commitment, and a sense of adventure to "stretch" a bit as a professional—to go into "uncharted" territory and to acknowledge some uncertainty and lack of clarity about what is going to happen and how the experience will unfold as the group develops into a team. When a new member joins an existing IHCT, there is also lack of clarity about how the new member will change the team and what he or she will contribute to it. IHCT members in these contexts become both teacher and learner. They can teach each other about their own unique perspectives as professionals and the roles they play. Additionally, they can learn from each other about different dimensions represented in the varied health care professions and how they can incorporate powerful insights from other disciplines into their own professional practice to make themselves better clinicians.

The Clinical Team That Would Not Be a Learning Team

An educational consultant was hired to work with what was essentially a multidisciplinary clinical team in a large health care system. The team was multidisciplinary in the sense that the members did not work in an interconnected fashion; rather, they made "parallel" contributions to the team. They did not really work at the higher level of understanding each other's discipline that we associate with the interdisciplinary level of functioning.

The consultant was called in by the hospital administration to provide "educational" training for this team. This training included assessments of the perception of different member's roles on the team, IHCT theory and practice, and general insights into team functioning based on current research. Not surprisingly, the consultant was met with a set of hostile reactions. "We're too busy with our heavy clinical load to take time for this," "We already know all this—it is a waste of time with all the patients we are responsible for," and "We don't know why you are here—were you brought in by the administration as a 'spy' because they think that something is wrong with our team?"

These reactions revealed a fundamental problem with this team and a basic insight into healthy IHCTs. The problem was that these clinicians were too busy with their work to learn—to learn more about teamwork and to learn from and about each other. The important insight to be gained from this experience is that teamwork is fundamentally a learning—rather than a clinical—activity. As such, the team needs time to reflect on what it is learning, why it is learning, and how to improve its learning. These insights are based on experiential learning theory.

WHAT IS EXPERIENTIAL LEARNING?

Elements of the Learning Cycle

Learning is best conceived of as a process, not a product or an outcome. As such, it stands in contrast with the major thrust of higher education in general, with which most students and practicing health care professionals are familiar. In the common understanding of learning, students or trainees master a particular body of knowledge that exists "out there," and they demonstrate their acquisition of this knowledge by testing. In this model, learning is based on outcomes: The instructor is the depositor, and students the recipients of knowledge deposits. In contrast, learning conceived of as a process suggests that the insights and skills acquired by participants in an experience are the learning. For example, we have had students in an IHCT course who thought that the required readings were the most important part of the course. By mid-semester, however, these students realized that the problems they encountered in actually trying to work together and the solutions they developed for these problems were the real learning.

Experiential learning is a conflict-filled process, and out of this conflict comes the development of genuine insight and skill. Part of this conflict is due to the fact that different individuals or health care professionals learn through different types of interaction with the world about them. According to experiential learning theory,[1] these styles exist along two polarities: concrete experience ("feeling") versus abstract conceptualization ("thinking"), and active experimentation ("doing") versus reflective observation ("watching"):

1. *Concrete experience* (CE) emphasizes personal involvement with people in everyday situations. Greater reliance is placed on sensitivity to feelings and people than on a systematic approach to problems and situations.

2. *Abstract conceptualization* (AC) involves using logic and ideas, rather than feelings, to understand situations. Systematic planning and the development of ideas and theories are used to solve problems.

3. *Active experimentation* (AE) connotes influencing or changing situations. It involves a practical approach to "what really works," or "what gets the job done," rather than simply watching a situation.

4. *Reflective observation* (RO) involves a careful observation before making a judgment, including examining a situation from various points of view. Patience, objectivity, and careful judgment are valued, not necessarily the taking of concrete action.

Individuals may use these various learning styles in different situations; and choosing which style or styles to use in a particular setting creates tension and conflict. Importantly, however, this structure represents the intrinsic nature of learning as a process incorporating all these elements. Learners must be able to involve themselves fully in new experiences (CE), be able to reflect on and observe their experiences from different perspectives (RO), create concepts that integrate their observations into logical theories (AC), and be able to use these theories to make decisions and to solve problems (AE). In the process of learning, one moves successively through these modes, creating a learning cycle. Learning involves the integration of all these phases: feeling, watching, thinking, and doing.

The four elements will be used at various points by the different participants on an IHCT, accounting for differing perceptions of the significance of the team-building experience. Indeed, different professions represented on a team may have different preferred learning styles, the result either of self-selection into professional fields of study or of the professional socialization process itself. For example, research suggests that medicine is more concrete and social work more abstract, whereas both medicine and social work are more active than nursing—which is more reflective.[2] This may partially explain why in a study by Drinka, social workers and psychiatrists were the disciplines most apt to take on the difficult team role of process analyzer.[3]

There is evidence that members of an IHCT use different learning elements for different tasks, and that they perceive some tasks as needing more expertise and therefore as more difficult than others.[4] Even experienced health care providers may appear to overuse "RO" for tasks they are not prepared to perform and that they perceive as very difficult (e.g., the leadership roles of "judge" and "process analyzer" may be quite difficult for many health care providers). Additional circumstances like having to teach a health care professional from another discipline adds to the difficulty of certain categories of tasks. The willingness to assume and teach team tasks may co-vary with the status of the health care worker a member engages with and the type of task at hand. One study demonstrated this to be the case with team members teaching other members to assume leadership (see Table 8.1).[5] In this study, even some seasoned team members engaged in RO for 3 years before assuming leadership tasks that they perceived as difficult. Other team members never assumed certain leadership tasks.

Table 8.1
Perceived Level of Expertise Required for Teaching Team Members
to Assume Leadership

Persons taught	Clinical administrative tasks	Socio-emotional support	Questioning clinical treatment issues	Process analyzing/ counseling
Staff from other profession	moderate	moderate	high	high
Staff from same profession	moderate	moderate	high	high
Student from other profession	low	low	high	high
Student from same profession	low	low	moderate	moderate

The experiential learning cycle is not static; rather, it results in a dynamic process of learning that is directional, with forward movement toward the acquisition of skills and knowledge. This suggests that as an IHCT develops higher levels of function and cohesion, it also increasingly becomes a learning team. Its members face conflicts and problems that are overcome and integrated into a higher level of team functioning. Learning occurs in response to the situations and circumstances in which the team finds itself, and individual members' learning becomes increasingly a function of the social environment of the team. That is, learning becomes less and less a solitary activity, and more and more one that is mediated by the group and the team context. These insights are illustrated in the words of a physician as she reflects on her learning process on an IHCT. She speaks of the length of time for the learning to occur, the importance of members transmitting team history, and the gradual process of becoming ready to learn.

A Physician's View of Learning

No [the didactics] didn't sink in at all. You know when I really started to understand the team? I came in September and I did 3 months of Evaluation Unit and then 3 months of research. On the Evaluation Unit I was so caught up with trying to get my feet on the ground trying to figure out who [the patient] was appropriate and who wasn't. . . . I didn't know about all of the team resources that would have helped me out. . . . You tend to go to the other fellows [physicians]—well you ask another fellow who is appropriate. . . . And then I did 3 months of research and was totally not involved. Then finally that spring I did home care and it all started to click, which is probably why I have this feeling about home care that it is the greatest thing because all of a sudden it all made sense. . . .

Let me start with some history. . . . I had gotten involved in changing the interdisciplinary treatment plan and the flow sheet but it wasn't 'til I realized what some of the history was that I was able to see that some of the things that I was recommending as changes had already been tried or hadn't worked or had already gone through these various phases. . . . I think initially I thought I did more than I realized. I really didn't when I realized what some of the total history was and I think what happened was that [another physician] had really taken it over and then we started talking about it and started working together, then I realized that both of us are missing out on things that had already been done and that's when I started to talk to one of the nurses more who is so intimately involved with it and has been for so much longer than either the other physician or I had been. I realized that these great contributions that we were making, that we just didn't have enough experience to be able to make them, which is when in getting the input of [two long-term team members] it became clearer that we could both sit at our computers and come up with these great treatment plans but the fact was that we weren't going to be able to do it without significant input from these people who had been here longer and who had been through all of the other changes. . . . You have to be ready to learn or to hear what is said. When I was working on the Evaluation Unit's policy manual I thought my God I wish someone had shown this to me or told me it existed when I started out on the Evaluation Unit because I had so many questions and I didn't know what to do or what the policies were or anything like that. And the social worker said, if we had handed this to you . . . and she is right, I wouldn't have read it.

The Social Context for Interdisciplinary Learning

Learning on IHCTs is a socially mediated process. This means that the learning is based on insights gained by interactions and shared experiences with others. This approach to understanding learning is part of a larger collaborative or cooperative learning movement in the United States, which emphasizes the importance of community—not individualism—in learning. The sense of community, of belonging to a group larger than oneself, is the foundation of knowledge creation itself. In this view, as in the general view of learning as based fundamentally on experience, knowledge is not something simply to be transmitted from teacher to student (the "banking" model). Rather, knowledge is created in the collaborative interchange; it is discovered in the process of experiencing interaction among the members of the team. Thus, the outcome of the educational process is more than the sum of its individual contributors, and the learning team or collaborative is the source of new knowledge and insights.

Learning on IHCTs consists of four fundamental dimensions: (a) individual skills as they relate to the team, (b) the understanding of the nature of professional roles and knowledge, (c) team process and skills, and (d) an understanding of how the team relates to the organization. Individual skills relate to the intelligence, experience, communication, and leadership skills that an individual brings to the team. These may or may not fit with the team's culture. Members' willingness to evaluate the skills they bring to a team and the relevance of these skills for the team are important. However, members' willingness to improve their skills is even more critical.

The second area of learning relates to an understanding by individual IHCT members of the roles and knowledge base of their own and other health professions. In this sense, members of the team learn from each other about what each health profession is and does. It is always revealing to participate in an IHCT training program and discover how many health care professionals really do not know what other health professions do. This knowledge is not part of their training; it is acquired by actually working closely with different professions, preferably in an interdisciplinary, collaborative setting. Participants come to understand that the knowledge they possess has been acquired by socialization within the confines of their own professional culture and disciplinary training, and that this knowledge has both great power and severe limitations. For the first time, IHCT members become consciously aware of how knowledge is generated, used, and transmitted in professional practice—and, more importantly, how understanding and interpretation of knowledge differ among various health professions. This awareness can best be attained in a teamwork setting in which the emergence of interdisciplinary relationships mediates cognitive development.

The third area of learning, team process, consists of basic small group and teamwork skills that some members may already have. Others will need to acquire them. However, it is critical that a new team address these issues as it gains collective experience. Dealing with conflict and communication problems, power and authority, and leadership concerns are the types of issues in this category. For a team to move to higher levels of development and maturity, these concerns will have to be dealt with as a team. Otherwise, the team may stagnate and become fixated at a particular level of development because it is unwilling or unable to deal with problems arising in these areas. This type of learning may require the assistance of an outside team process consultant or a mentoring team, who can assist the group in overcoming barriers to effective teamwork and in achieving the higher levels of functional integration that characterize a true team. Trainees and new team members to existing teams will have to gain this experience in a different way (i.e., they will have to rely on mentors and an interactive educational process with existing team members).

A fourth dimension of learning on an IHCT is that of the team's relationship to the organization. This is the dimension of learning that is most often neglected by academic institutions and by IHCTs. It is also the dimension that health care providers most want to ignore. However, if we are going to change the way that health care is practiced so that patients are treated holistically, organizational leaders must learn what IHCTs are, how they differ from their existing concepts of teams, how to work with members of IHCTs, and how to measure the effects of teamwork. Conversely, members of IHCTs must learn how to work with the stakeholders in the systems in which they operate. If different health care professionals come from different planets, administrators of health care come from another solar system. These gaps in understanding can be bridged by mutual listening and by dialogue. That dialogue is unlikely to occur as part of basic training, and thus will have to occur as a result of active engagement during ongoing team development.

Charting Interdisciplinary Teamwork Learning

Insights into the nature of teamwork learning can be gained by the use of journaling—an instructional method requiring the keeping of a personal diary that includes a description both of "what happened" and of "what it means." We have taught a course on teamwork in which students are required to design, develop, and deliver a health promotion workshop program for older adults in the community. They are also asked to maintain a written journal chronicling their personal thoughts regarding the experiences encountered as part of the IHCT. One of the strengths of the use of journaling is that it enables the teamwork instructor to look at the personal responses and reactions of different members of the team over the course of the learning experience—to assess their progression from being simply a team "member" to becoming a team "player."

The written journal we have used is based on the work of Schatzman and Strauss, which emphasizes the use of the journal as a written record of "learning as a developmental dialogue."[6] In this approach, which is consistent with conceptualizing learning as experience, learning is conceived of as an interactional, developmental process of discovery, in which reflection and the development of meaning are central. The entries in this journal entail three types of notes, around which the observer organizes "packages" of material. These are observational notes (ONs), theoretical notes (TNs), and methodological notes (MNs).

ONs are statements about events experienced through watching and listening, but they contain as little interpretive material as possible. Included are the basic "who, what, where, when, and how" of people's activities, with each note a discrete event or unit. Conversation or dialogue may be included, particularly exchanges between persons that have significance for the observer.

In contrast, TNs represent the observer's attempt to make sense or meaning of what has been seen or heard, including the use of concepts or theories that may aid in this process. These notes include the development of hypotheses and interpretations to be noted, stored, and re-evaluated against past and future entries.

Finally, MNs are statements that act as instructions, reminders, and notes to the observer, a kind of written bulletin board for keeping the observational or reflective process on track. In a sense, MNs serve as mirrors through which the observer thinks about the very process in which he or she is engaged.

The entries that follow are taken from the actual journal of one student in our teamwork course. The types of team learning that are reflected in it relate to the following areas: skills development in communication and conflict management; greater clarity on one's own professional role and how it relates to those of other professions; greater willingness to rely on input and assistance of others on the IHCT; enhanced professional judgment and perspective on the meaning of different professions and their interrelationships; improved sense of self-confidence as a professional vis-à-vis others; and appreciation for the value of teamwork.

Sample Entries from Student Journal: Dietetics Undergraduate

September 15

ON   Today I read the research article titled "A Service/Learning Model for Interdisciplinary Teamwork in Health and Aging."

TN   I realized in order to provide the maximum care to my patients, it is best to seek other health care providers' advice. My own viewpoint is only that, one way of seeing the whole picture, or in that matter only a part of the picture. Health care providers need to work hand in hand in order to deliver information far above [what] one professional could achieve individually.

October 4

ON   The five of us met . . . to draw up an assessment list of our population, for the six workshops we will be delivering to the senior center.

TN   As we all took turns suggesting workshop topics, it really hit me how each topic can really be interrelated into all of our major fields of study. Each topic can be expanded and interpreted by all five of us in different lights. Each topic can be developed in many ways depending on who is viewing the topic.

MN   I must remember to be aware of the "team" and the other "players" and the resources they can help supply rather than attempt to try and do everything myself.

October 18

ON   The topic of class was learning, but more specifically adult learning, since [older adults] are the target audience.

TN   A teamwork approach is probably the most well-rounded strategy in the learning process. We as a "team" bring in a variety of skills into each situation, so together [we] can promote optimal learning.

MN   I think the team should keep in mind that learning is a process, not an outcome. We must remember we are facilitators for communication and must let our audience be the active participants.

October 25

ON   The idea of conflict and its effect on the team was discussed.

TN   Conflict is healthy and allows the group to grow, just by the necessity of dealing with the problem at hand. Conflict is only negative when it is ignored. I had a conflict with the rest of the team when they insisted I participate in the workshop on vitamins. I did not believe in the topic, and the last thing I wanted to do was participate in such a workshop. The end result was that I will be an active participant because the team showed me how I can play a positive role in the situation. I now see how important it is for open communication within the team. As a result, I also feel a stronger commitment to the team.

MN   We must remember that each discipline's role is equally important. Furthermore, whether we agree or disagree with individual topics, we should not avoid these situations but use them as educational opportunities. We as a "team" need to keep in mind that these types of conflicts are not bad, but beneficial for allowing the team to grow. If ignored, a breakdown of the whole team could result.

October 30

ON   I gathered final thoughts for my paper.

ON   Today, I drew many conclusions concerning the power of interdisciplinary teams, which was the title for my first reaction paper. I also combined many supporting examples when possible.

TN   Although I have been keeping a journal frequently through the semester, I never realized how strong a team was until I wrote my paper. The paper helped organize my thoughts and made it very clear to me that there is tremendous power in an interdisciplinary team.

MN   Now that I've written my paper, I will remember the role of an interdisciplinary team. I know how I can help make positive changes in other people's lives, by helping them to help themselves. I am now much more confident in my position as a team member and this will be beneficial to the target audience.

November 1

ON   I read an article . . . which was also discussed in class. . . . The article emphasized knowledge as the basis of professions, and the importance of understanding cognitive maps between each discipline.

TN   Earlier this semester I learned that each discipline might interpret the same word quite differently, now this article really brings out the necessity to understand how other disciplines can "see" things differently. . . . I realize now how two different disciplines may observe the same thing two very different ways. We as a team need to be aware of each other's cognitive maps, so we will be clear and avoid any confusion on what is being observed. Each member will become more well rounded and acquire a broader knowledge base through a team experience, in my opinion.

November 8

ON   This afternoon I met with [the nursing student] to prepare and made some final decisions for our workshop.

TN   I think it is interesting how two people who may not have anything else in common but this class can work so well together to reach the common goal . . . of patient welfare.

MN   It seems important to remember what our common goal is, because that helps bring the members together and it provides an aim for the team to focus on, and not get confused with personal objectives.

November 30

ON   [The psychology student] and I met this evening . . . to expand on our past ideas for the [next] workshop. This meeting went a lot smoother than our first.

MN   It is important to remember that planning and developing ideas takes time and we should not be discouraged if at first we do not reach our desired outcome. In addition, we must also learn it is okay to depend on each other for support and encouragement because after all we are all part of the same "team."

December 6

ON   Today's class . . . [is] going to be our last official class meeting.

ON [The pharmacy student and I] worked on our final plans for the workshop . . . on vitamins.

TN I was amazed to see how much I have changed over the semester. I am more confident in my role as a Dietitian, and have increased my sense of security of being an active member of this team. I feel the personal attention I have received . . . and the team has helped to contribute to the positive behavior changes that I have encountered.

MN I should keep in mind that I have a lot of knowledge on this subject, and should voice the facts, and not be afraid that some people may disagree. This will be my chance to test the confidence that I have gained this semester.

December 9

ON [The pharmacy student] and I met . . . today at [the site] to perform the vitamin workshop.

TN Well, the workshop was a success. The audience was very receptive to our information. . . . Once we started the workshop my anxiety was lessened, and I felt good. I no longer felt any conflict about the situation.

MN We must remember that conflicts are helpful in allowing the team to grow. They are beneficial, if they are properly addressed. The problem arises when they are ignored, and a gradual breakdown of the whole team occurs. Our team has been alert and has not let conflicts bring us down. We in fact became stronger as a result of them.

From this journal is evident the kind of progress that the student has made in understanding teamwork, her role on the IHCT, and—perhaps most importantly—how the team member role can strengthen her own work as a health care professional. The journal revealed the kinds of transformations in thinking and behavior that were a direct result of the social (i.e., interdisciplinary) learning environment of the teamwork course.

IMPLICATIONS OF CONCEPTUALIZING TEAMWORK AS A FORM OF EXPERIENTIAL LEARNING

There are several important implications of conceptualizing teamwork and the process of becoming an IHCT as a form of experiential learning. These follow from a corollary of the principle that all learning is grounded in experience: namely, that all learning is really relearning. As Kolb, a major theorist in experiential learning, stated:

The fact that learning is a continuous process grounded in experience has important educational implications. Put simply, it implies that all learning is relearning. . . . [O]ne's job as an educator is not only to implant new ideas but also to dispose of or modify old ones. In many cases, resistance to new ideas stems from their conflict with old beliefs that are inconsistent with them. If the education process begins by bringing out the learner's beliefs and theories, examining and testing them, and then integrating the new, more refined ideas into the person's belief systems, the learning process will be facilitated.[7]

The implications of this perspective for education and training in interdisciplinary teamwork fall into the following categories: specifying learning objectives, the problem of timing, the role of the instructor, instructional methods, and the importance of context.

Specifying Learning Objectives

Most academic courses and educational workshops are expected to state clearly what the students or trainees should know or be able to do following the completion of the experience. However, in the field of interdisciplinary teamwork, we often seem to fall short of clearly articulating what should be the type of learning outcomes associated with a course or a workshop. At the most basic level, is the purpose simply to introduce the participant to the main ideas and concepts in teamwork, as well as to some basic principles related to team functioning and dynamics? This level could be considered a type of educational "enrichment"—an interesting exposure to the ideas, but not one that is sufficient to make any meaningful change in actual clinical behavior.

Or, at a more advanced level, is the objective to inculcate the actual group skills in communication and conflict management needed for successful teams, as well as the understanding of the cognitive and value maps of different participating health professions? If so, this type of outcome requires more in-depth exposure and training commitment, with the opportunity to practice in field settings, perhaps as a member of an actual IHCT. Many current models of training seem to fall into this category, in which students in an academic course for a semester or actual practicing professionals at a clinical site are expected to develop a fairly extensive knowledge and skills base in teamwork.

Or, is the purpose of interdisciplinary education to train the next generation of team leaders who will provide the leadership needed to carry forward the knowledge and skills needed for successful IHCTs in health care organizations? Here, the training needed would probably be over a period of several months or even years, suggesting a major commitment from the learner to the field of teamwork and to acquiring the level of knowledge and skills necessary to truly master the multiple facets of clinical and educational theory and practice in the field.

Each of these sets of objectives connotes very different levels of exposure to teamwork, resources needed to support them, and commitment from the trainee. In reality, we need all of these levels of education, and some in-between, to provide an adequate basis for IHCTs in the future. We may think of this as "basic," "intermediate," and "advanced" training—the equivalent of introductory, middle-level, and advanced courses—or different levels of professional certification in a specific field.

Interdisciplinary Practice as a Jazz Ensemble:
An Instructional Metaphor

Effective interdisciplinary teamwork may be likened to a jazz ensemble. Jazz does not rely on a written score, nor is there usually a conductor. Rather, the theme is passed from one musician to another; improvisation is used freely, but there is a general pattern and structure to the music. The contributions of different instruments to the overall richness of the music are valued; missing "voices" of absent instruments stand out and are apparent in the sound of the music.

Similarly, in an effectively functioning IHCT there may be flexible leadership, as the clinical cases and issues may change and necessitate different disciplines taking the lead. The voices of different disciplines are important to the overall mission and effectiveness of the team—their absence may make the work of the team more difficult or less efficient. The pattern of communication among the team members is open and dynamic: Members may anticipate what others will say or what they are thinking, and they take these into account as they make their own contributions to furthering the team's mission. Role flexibility and interconnected communication lead to an appreciation of teamwork as an artform!

The Problem of Timing

The issue of the timing of interdisciplinary teamwork learning relates more to academic educational settings than clinical training for currently practicing health care professionals. This problem is based on the question of when is the optimal time for students to participate in teamwork experiences in a way that builds their familiarity with and expertise in IHCTs. Educators need to provide both strong disciplinary instruction and interdisciplinary teamwork opportunities for health professions students and current professionals to learn the joys and challenges of working together. This must be done in a parallel and dialectical way that shapes and enhances skills in both these areas.

For example, as students gain greater mastery of their own, unique professional identity they need to be introduced to opportunities for working together in IHCTs in clinical practice settings. Some proficiency in the basic knowledge and skill of each discipline is necessary for the students at least to know "what part they have," but waiting until they have graduated before giving them the opportunity to collaborate is a mistake. Rather, gradual and graduated opportunities—and time for reflection on the process of working and learning together—are essential ingredients of effective instruction. This suggests that teamwork needs to be integrated, stepwise, into existing curricula, with the degree of exposure in proportion to the students' emerging sense of professional identity and ability to consider perspectives other than their own.

Similarly, continuing education opportunities can be provided in support of currently practicing professionals wanting more training in teamwork and collaborative skills. This could take the form of general workshops on the knowledge and skills necessary for effective team-building, as well as more individualized team development and process consultation. In most cases, currently practicing professionals have little background or training in teamwork, yet they are often thrust into situations where they are expected to work as part of an IHCT. As has been pointed out before, simply putting nice people together does not make them a team!

The Role of the Instructor

The role of the instructor in interdisciplinary teamwork learning also merits some thought. In a fundamental sense, members of IHCTs are both learners and teachers. They learn from one another and they teach each other about the roles, knowledge, and values of different health professions. However, teaching each other across disciplines is not necessarily an easy task, as the ability to teach must be learned and the willingness to teach must be acquired. All team members will not be willing to teach or mentor in all team areas. On well-functioning IHCTs, team members learn as a group about what it takes to work together effectively, about the requisite skills needed to be a good team player. As we have said, this learning is based on the experience itself of working together, and it cannot be "taught" in the usual way we think of teaching by an instructor.

This insight raises another important question: What is the appropriate role for the instructor in an IHCT course or workshop? If the experience is the learning, then what is the appropriate role for the teacher? As Kolb suggested, the role of the educator is not only to present new ideas, but also to address the old ones that may impede the acquisition of the new. In this sense, the metaphor of the "coach" is instructive. The coach must be able to assess the needs of his or her protégé in terms of the steps that must be taken to reach the objective of being a team player. This assessment requires an examination of both where one is coming from or where one is, and where one should be. Importantly, the path is clear only to those who have already reached this stage, and the coach must provide the knowledge and instill the confidence needed for the student or trainee to proceed, step by step, along the path of becoming resocialized as a team player. Schön also used the metaphor of coaching in his discussion of the acquisition of professional artistry, quoting from the work of John Dewey:

The student cannot be *taught* what he needs to know, but he can be *coached*: "He has to *see* on his own behalf and in his own way the relations between means and methods employed and results achieved. Nobody else can see for him, and he can't see just by being 'told,' although the right kind of telling may guide his seeing and thus help him see what he needs to see."[8]

Coaching may be facilitated by the use of such learning techniques as the journal, which provides a window into the team participants' inner thoughts and reactions to the challenge of becoming a team player, essential information for the coach to have to provide effective guidance and advice. The journal may reveal inner conflicts, questions, and thought processes on the part of an individual that stand in the way of IHCT formation; similarly, it allows the coach or instructor to see where the members are and where they need to be for the team to function effectively as a unit.

Instructional Methods

Experiential learning opportunities at clinical sites where multiple professions work together collaboratively would be ideal settings for this type of instruction, provided they are supported by a course or seminar structure that affords students the time and opportunity to reflect on their experiences in working together. Various models of actual courses developed along these lines have been described in the gerontological and geriatric educational literature, and similar approaches are available in other fields.[9]

Additionally, the development of service-learning model courses, in which students participate in community-based (rather than clinical) programs, provides a new opportunity to develop collaborative skills in settings that will be increasingly important as health interventions move out of traditional institutional contexts into this broader arena.[10] The emerging national movement combining service-learning programs and community-academic partnerships is a recognition of the importance of these basic concepts.[11]

Finally, the development of structured case studies (as used in problem-based learning methods) gives students the opportunity to identify and address the multifaceted health problems of certain types of patients. If carefully constructed to embody the need for many disciplines to be involved in team care, such cases would be an excellent opportunity for participants with different backgrounds to work together. Importantly, however, these instructional methods need to be specifically developed to require truly interdisciplinary collaboration—with intersecting patterns of disciplinary communication—rather than the more parallel lines that typify multidisciplinary training.

This educational process may be thought of as one of "dual socialization," in which students develop identities of both "individual professional" and "team player." These two processes complement each other, as students only really learn "who they are" when they have to define themselves and their professional focus in the context of others. This includes an assessment of who may overlap with them in some areas and share a common identity, or be complementary to them in other important dimensions of clinical practice. Indeed, theories of identity formation during the period of adolescence and young adulthood emphasize the importance of a "moratorium" period when the individual can "try on" different identities before determining the "right one" for him or her. Similarly, in the process of coming to know "who I am" as a physician, nurse, social worker, occupational or physical therapist, pharmacist, or dietitian, exposure to a range of different identities may ultimately lead to a more reflective and confident professional. This professional is one who has "chosen" his or her identity in a way that recognizes both the importance of one's own profession and the necessity of valuing the diversity of others in the delivery of clinical care.

Teamwork Instruction as Music Lessons and Band or Orchestra

The need for both disciplinary and interdisciplinary training for students in the health professions can be compared to music instruction—a metaphor introduced earlier in the comparison of an effective IHCT with a jazz ensemble.

Although students take lessons individually on their own instrument, they also play together in bands or orchestras. This "parallel" instruction is seen as essential for the development of individual expertise and skill on the instrument, as well as for the ability to play together and to make the more pleasing sounds that come from instruments raising their "voices" collectively in a great work of music.

We would probably not think of separating these two forms of instruction; they are seen as complementary and an integral part of the unified experience of playing a musical instrument. Similarly, we must come to think of good health professional education as incorporating both discipline-specific teaching and interdisciplinary practice opportunities.

The Importance of Context

In our experience, the setting in which an IHCT operates or for which its members are being trained is seldom addressed in terms of educational implications. However, the primary mission of the team, based in part on the organizational context in which it operates, is important to its mission, focus, and dynamics. For example, an IHCT in an acute care setting may have a very different set of objectives from one working with persons living in the community. A hospital provides a much more structured and defined setting than a community, with corresponding implications for the perceived roles of different members of the IHCT and how they interpret their involvement on it.

Similarly, the type of experiences encountered by the IHCT and its members will affect the ways they learn from each other—experiences that may reinforce traditional roles or call into question the roles for which students or trainees were prepared. For example, a hospital context may simply reinforce team members' perceptions of their roles in the fairly typical setting afforded by an acute care model. In contrast, a community-based team that encounters health problems "where people live everyday" may be forced to question its fundamental assumptions about the underlying causes of health problems and their solutions. The "mission" of such a team may become increasingly "psychosocial" and much less "biomedical," for example. Such a shift has implications for how the team members interpret and understand their own unique roles.

Instructors seldom take these types of differences into account, yet these differences also have implications for how instructors perceive their roles. For example, the educator in the hospital-based setting may have a much more traditional role in this controlled learning environment than the relatively more unpredictable setting of the community—where "anything can happen." In the former context, the role of educator may be more akin to the standard "teacher" role, whereas in the latter it may be closer to that of a "facilitator" who encourages students to see and experience things differently. Service-learning models of education, for example, emphasize a much less-structured and more supportive role for the instructor than traditional, classroom, or didactic methods.

A final word about two additional areas of "learning and teaching" that are relevant to IHCTs: teaching the patient to participate in the team process, and teaching the organization about teamwork. Teaching the patient deals with the issue of how to involve the patient and the family more completely in the process of defining the health "problem" and identifying potential "solutions" to it. Some health care professionals advocate very strongly for patient involvement in the team—indeed, some argue that the patient should be the team leader. Others suggest that this is not practical. Overall, however, most observers agree that patients must know more about how to relate to an IHCT and develop an understanding of what the team is and what it is not. In this respect, IHCTs are similar to other kinds of service teams—such as those in special education—where there may be a strong focus on the family and its involvement in the team's work.[12] At the very least, patients and their families should be taught about what the team is, what to expect from it, and how the team members work together to share their expertise to improve patient outcomes. How this information is taught should be up to the IHCT itself to discuss and decide, much as it would collaborate on other issues of clinical concern.

Teaching the organization about teamwork concerns the responsibility of team members to educate their respective health care organizations (including administrators) about how IHCTs operate, what they need to do their work well, and why teams are better than solo practitioners in addressing health problems with multiple and complicated features. Just as it is important to teach patients, it is also important for members of IHCTs to teach other clinicians within the organization how to interact with the team and what they can expect from the team. It is a mistake for team members to believe that the organization will automatically notice the team's clinical successes. If teams establish mechanisms to accept feedback on their operation (e.g., from clinical outcome data, health care clinicians, and administrators who are external to the team), the team can use this information to improve its service to the organization in general. Sharing these improvement examples can be an effective mechanism for teaching the organization about teamwork. All team members can assume the leadership task of gathering clinical examples concerning how the team helped patients in ways that a solo practitioner or a multidisciplinary team could not. On a regular basis, a formal team leader can perform the task of relating the best case examples and other improvement data to administrators. This formal leader can also suggest innovative ways to view and measure clinical team outcomes.

SUMMARY

In summary, several variables create a unique learning and teaching context in teamwork. Indeed, teams and teamwork tend to alter dramatically our usual conceptions of education and clinical practice, of teaching and learning. They force us to adopt new interpretations of what it means to be teacher or student, participant or observer, and practice-oriented or theory-based. Experiential learning, the core of genuine understanding of team development as learning, suggests that learning is a cycle of experiencing and thinking, intervening and reflecting. If we think of the team as a self-directed learning unit, then we must consider that all of these activities are essential to the learning process. In reality, IHCTs see their mission primarily as one of "doing," rather than as one of "learning." Changing this conception is the primary task of educators who want both to train health professionals to work together and to foster lifelong learning at the same time.

NOTES

1. Kolb, D. A. (1984). *Experiential learning*. Englewood Cliffs, NJ: Prentice-Hall.

2. Ibid.

3. Drinka, T.J.K. (1991). A case study of leadership on a long term interdisciplinary health care team (Doctoral dissertation, University of Wisconsin-Madison, 1990). *Dissertation Abstracts* International, *51:11*, 3599A.

4. Ibid.

5. Ibid.

6. Schatzman, L., & Strauss, A. (1973). *Field research: Strategies for a natural sociology*. Englewood Cliffs, NJ: Prentice-Hall.

7. Kolb, *Experiential learning*, p. 28.

8. Schön, D. A. (1987). *Educating the reflective practitioner*. San Francisco, CA: Jossey-Bass, p. 17.

9. Allen, R. M., Koch, M. L., & Williams, J. D. (1984). An interdisciplinary gerontology elective for allied health students. *Gerontology & Geriatrics Education, 4*(4), 85–90; Bennett, R., & Miller, P. (1987). Interdisciplinary approach to graduate health sciences education in geriatrics and gerontology. In G. Lessnoff-Caravaglia (Ed.), *Handbook of applied gerontology* (pp. 155–170). New York: Human Sciences Press; Kappelman, M. M., Bartnick, L. A., Cahn, B., & Rapoport, M. I. (1981). A non-traditional geriatric teaching model: Interprofessional service/education sites. *Journal of Medical Education, 56*, 467–477; Morrissey, S., Moore, S., Cox, G., Queiro-Tajalli, I., & Martz, B. L. (1989). Building interdisciplinary teams in gerontological education. *Educational Gerontology, 15*, 385–394.

10. Clark, P. G., Spence, D. L., & Sheehan, J. L. (1986). A service/learning model for interdisciplinary teamwork in health and aging. *Gerontology & Geriatrics Education, 6*(4), 3–16.

11. Clark, P. G. (1999). Service-learning education in community-academic partnerships: Implications for interdisciplinary geriatric training in the health professions. *Educational Gerontology, 25*, 641–660.

12. Clark, P. G. (1996). Learning from education: What the teamwork literature in special education can teach gerontologists about team training and development. *Educational Gerontology, 22*, 387–410.

Bibliography

Abramson, M. (1984). Collective responsibility in interdisciplinary collaboration: An ethical perspective for social workers. *Social Work in Health Care, 10*(1), 35–43.

Allen, R. M., Koch, M. L., & Williams, J. D. (1984). An interdisciplinary gerontology elective for allied health students. *Gerontology & Geriatrics Education, 4*(4), 85–90.

Anderson, O., & Gevitz, N. (1983). The general hospital: A social and historical perspective. In D. Mechanic (Ed.), *Handbook of health, health care, and the health professions* (pp. 305–317). New York: The Free Press.

Andre, J. (1992). Learning to see: Moral growth during medical training. *Journal of Medical Ethics, 18*, 148–152.

Argyris, C. (1982). *Reasoning, learning, and action: Individual and organizational.* San Francisco: Jossey-Bass.

Argyris, C., Putnam, R., & Smith, D. M. (1987). *Action science.* San Francisco: Jossey-Bass.

Aumann, G.M.-E., & Cole, T. R. (1991). In whose voice? Composing a lifesong collaboratively. *The Journal of Clinical Ethics, 2*, 45–49.

Baldwin, D. C. (1996). Some historical notes on interdisciplinary and interprofessional education and practice in health care in the USA. *Journal of Interprofessional Care, 10*, 173–187.

Bales, R. F., & Slater, P. (1955). Role differentiation in small social groups. In T. Parsons, R. F. Bales, & E. A. Shils (Eds.), *Family, socialisation and interaction process* (pp. 259–306). Glencoe, IL: The Free Press.

Bass, B. M. (1990). *Bass and Stogdill's handbook of leadership: Theory, research and managerial applications* (3rd ed.). New York: The Free Press.

Bass, B. M., Waldman, D. A., Avolio, B. J., & Bebb, M. (1987). Transformational leadership and the falling dominoes effect. *Group and Organization Studies, 12*, 73–87.

Beckhouse, L. S., Tanur, J., Weiler, J., & Weinstein, E. (1975). And some men have leadership thrust upon them. *Journal of Personality and Social Psychology, 31*, 557–566.

Bennett, R., & Miller, P. (1987). Interdisciplinary approach to graduate health sciences education in geriatrics and gerontology. In G. Lessnoff-Caravaglia (Ed.), *Handbook of applied gerontology* (pp. 155–170). New York: Human Sciences Press.

Bennis, W. G. (1965). Theory and method in applying behavioral science to planned organizational change. *Journal of Applied Behavioral Science, 1*, 337–360.

Bennis, W., & Nanus, B. (1985). *Leaders: The strategies for taking charge*. New York: Harper & Row.

Bennis, W., & Townsend, R. (1995). *Reinventing leadership: Strategies to empower the organization*. New York: William Morrow.

Blake, R. R., & Mouton, J. S. (1964). *The managerial grid*. Houston: Gulf.

Bloom, S. W. (1979). Socialization for the physician's role: A review of some contributions of research to theory. In E. C. Shapiro & L. M. Lowenstein (Eds.), *Becoming a physician: Development of values and attitudes in medicine* (pp. 3–52). Cambridge, MA: Ballinger.

Bloom, S. W. (1989). The medical school as social organization: The sources of resistance to change. *Medical Education, 23*, 228–241.

Bolman, L. G., & Deal, T. E. (1984). *Modern approaches to understanding and managing organizations*. San Francisco: Jossey-Bass.

Burns, J. M. (1978). *Leadership*. New York: Harper & Row.

Calder, B.-J. (1977). An attribution theory of leadership. In B. M. Staw & G. R. Salancik (Eds.), *New directions in organizational behavior* (pp.179–204). Chicago: St. Clair Press.

Cannon-Bowers, J. A., Tannenbaum, S. I., Salas, E., & Volpe, C. E. (1995). Defining competencies and establishing team training requirements. In R. A. Guzzo, E. Salas, & Assoc. (Eds.), *Team effectiveness and decision making in organizations* (pp. 333–380). San Francisco: Jossey-Bass.

Cartwright, D., & Zander, A. (1968). *Group dynamics: Research and method* (3rd ed.). New York: Harper & Row.

Charatan, F. B., Foley, C. J., & Libow, L. S. (1985). The team approach to geriatric medicine. In R. Andres, E. L. Bierman, & W. R. Hazzard (Eds.), *Principles of geriatric medicine* (pp. 169–175). New York: McGraw-Hill.

Cherkasky, M. (1949). The Montefiore hospital home care program. *American Journal of Public Health, 39*, 163–166.

Clark, P. G. (1991). Toward a conceptual framework for developing interdisciplinary teams in gerontology: Cognitive and ethical dimensions. *Gerontology & Geriatrics Education, 12*(1), 79–96.

Clark, P. G. (1993). A typology of interdisciplinary education in gerontology and geriatrics: Are we really doing what we say we are? *Journal of Interprofessional Care, 7*, 217–227.

Clark, P. G. (1994). Learning on interdisciplinary gerontological teams: Instructional concepts and methods. *Educational Gerontology, 20*, 349–364.

Clark, P. G. (1994). Social, professional, and educational values on the interdisciplinary team: Implications for gerontological and geriatric education. *Educational Gerontology, 20*, 35–51.

Clark, P. G. (1995). Quality of life, values, and teamwork in geriatric care: Do we communicate what we mean? *The Gerontologist, 35*, 402–411.

Clark, P. G. (1996). Communication between provider and patient: Values, biography, and empowerment in clinical practice. *Ageing and Society, 16*, 747–774.

Clark, P. G. (1996). Learning from education: What the teamwork literature in special education can teach gerontologists about team training and development. *Educational Gerontology, 22*, 387–410.

Clark, P. G. (1997). Values in health care professional socialization: Implications for geriatric education in interdisciplinary teamwork. *The Gerontologist, 37*, 441–451.

Clark, P. G. (1999). Service-learning education in community-academic partnerships: Implications for interdisciplinary geriatric training in the health professions. *Educational Gerontology, 25*, 641–660.

Clark, P. G., Puxty, J., & Ross, L. G. (1997). An interdisciplinary geriatric team training institute: What can we learn by studying processes and outcomes? *Educational Gerontology, 23*, 725–744.

Clark, P. G., Spence, D. L., & Sheehan, J. L. (1986). A service/learning model for interdisciplinary teamwork in health and aging. *Gerontology & Geriatrics Education, 6*(4), 3–16.

Clark, P. G., Spence, D. L., & Sheehan, J. L. (1987). Challenges and barriers to interdisciplinary gerontological team training in the academic setting. *Gerontology & Geriatrics Education, 7*(3/4), 93–110.

Collaborating for change in health professions education. (1996). *Joint Commission Journal on Quality Improvement, 22*(3).

Counsell, S. R., Kennedy, R. D., Szwabo, P., Wadsworth, N. S., & Wohlgemuth, C. (1999). Curriculum recommendations for resident training in geriatrics interdisciplinary team care. *Journal of the American Geriatrics Society, 47*, 1145–1148.

Davidson, W.A.S. (1991). Metaphors of health and aging: Geriatrics as metaphor. In G. M. Kenyon, J. E. Birren, & J.J.F. Schroots (Eds.), *Metaphors of aging in science and the humanities* (pp. 173–184). New York: Springer.

Deisher, R. W. (1953). Use of the child health conference in the training of medical students. *Pediatrics, 11,* 538–543.

DeJong, G. (1984). Independent living: From social movement to analytic paradigm. In P. Marinelli & A. Dell (Eds.), *The psychological and social impact of physical disability* (pp. 39–64). New York: Springer.

Dill, A. (1993). Defining needs, defining systems: A critical analysis. *The Gerontologist, 33,* 453–460.

Drinka, T.J.K. (1987). Interdisciplinary health team and organizational development literature: An analysis of approaches to conflict recognition, resolution, and management. In M. L. Brunner & R. M. Casto (Eds.), *Interdisciplinary health team care: Proceedings of the eighth annual conference* (pp. 74–84). Columbus: School of Allied Medical Professions and Commission on Interprofessional Education and Practice, The Ohio State University.

Drinka, T.J.K. (1991). A case study of leadership on a long term interdisciplinary health care team (Doctoral dissertation, University of Wisconsin-Madison, 1990). *Dissertation Abstracts International, 51:11,* 3599A.

Drinka, T.J.K. (1991). Development and maintenance of an interdisciplinary health care team: A case study. *Gerontology & Geriatrics Education, 12*(1), 111–127.

Drinka, T.J.K. (1994). Interdisciplinary geriatric teams: Approaches to conflict as indicators of potential to model teamwork. *Educational Gerontology, 20,* 87–103.

Drinka, T.J.K. (1996). Applying learning from self-directed work teams in business to curriculum development for interdisciplinary geriatric teams. *Educational Gerontology, 22,* 433–450.

Drinka, T.J.K, & Miller, T. F. (1996). The health care team as metaphor: A preliminary study. *Journal of Allied Health, 25*(3), 245–261.

Drinka, T.J.K., Miller, T. F., & Goodman, B. M. (1996). Characterizing motivational styles of professionals who work on interdisciplinary healthcare teams. *Journal of Interprofessional Care, 10,* 51–61.

Drinka, T., & Ray, R. O. (1986). An investigation of power in an interdisciplinary health care team. *Gerontology & Geriatrics Education, 6*(3), 43–53.

Drinka, T.J.K., & Ray, R. O. (1992). Health care team ≠ Health care team. In J. R. Snyder (Ed.), *Proceedings of the fourteenth annual conference on interdisciplinary health care teams* (pp. 1–12). Indianapolis: School of Allied Health Sciences, Indiana University Medical Center.

Drinka, T.J.K., & Streim, J. E. (1994). Case studies from purgatory: Maladaptive behavior within geriatrics health care teams. *The Gerontologist, 34,* 541–547.

Dumaine, B. (1994, September 5). The trouble with teams. *Fortune,* 86–92.

Fagermoen, M. S. (1995). *The meaning of nurses' work: A descriptive study of values fundamental to professional identity in nursing.* Unpublished doctoral dissertation, the University of Rhode Island, Kingston.

Fasano, L. A., Muskin, P. R., & Sloan, R. P. (1993). The impact of medical education on students' perceptions of patients. *Academic Medicine, 68*(Suppl.), S43–S45.

Fisher, B. A. (1986). Leadership: When does the difference make a difference? In R. A. Hirakawa & M. S. Poole (Eds.), *Communication and group decision-making* (pp. 197–215). Beverly Hills: Sage.

Ford, C. V. (1983). *The somatizing disorders: Illness as a way of life.* New York: Elsevier Science Publications.

Foti, R. J., Fraser, S. L., & Lord, R. G. (1982). Effects of leadership labels and prototypes on perceptions of political leaders. *Journal of Applied Psychology, 67,* 326–333.

Furnham, A. (1988). Values and vocational choice: A study of value differences in medical, nursing, and psychology students. *Social Science and Medicine, 26,* 613–618.

Gadow, S. (1983). Frailty and strength: The dialectic in aging. *The Gerontologist, 23,* 144–147.

Garvin, D. A. (1993, July–August). Building a learning organization. *Harvard Business Review,* 78–91.

Gawande, A. (1998, March 30). No mistake. *The New Yorker,* 74–81.

Geller, G., Faden, R. R., & Levine, D. M. (1990). Tolerance for ambiguity among medical students: Implications for their selection, training, and practice. *Social Science and Medicine, 31,* 619–624.

Gilligan, C. (1982). *In a different voice: Psychological theory and women's development.* Cambridge, MA: Harvard University Press.

Ginzberg, E., & Ostow, M. (1997). Managed care—a look back and a look ahead. *New England Journal of Medicine, 336,* 1018–1020.

Graen, G., Novak, M. A., & Sommerkamp, P. (1982). The effects of leader–member exchange and job design on productivity and satisfaction: Testing a dual attachment model. *Organizational Behavior and Human Performance, 30,* 109–131.

Gramelspacher, G. P., Howell, J. D., & Young, M. J. (1986). Perceptions of ethical problems by nurses and doctors. *Archives of Internal Medicine, 146,* 577–578.

Hall, J. (1986). *Conflict management survey.* Woodlands, TX: Teleometrics International.

Hersey, P., & Blanchard, K. (1982). *Management of organizational behavior: Utilizing human resources* (4th ed.). Englewood Cliffs, NJ: Prentice-Hall.

Hollander, E. P. (1961). Some effects of perceived status on responses to innovative behavior. *Journal of Abnormal and Social Psychology, 63,* 247–250.

Hollander, E. P. (1964). *Leaders, groups and influence*. New York: Oxford University Press.

Hollander, E. P. (1979). Leadership and social exchange processes. In K. J. Gergen, M. S. Greenberg, & R. H. Willis (Eds.), *Social exchange: Advances in theory and research* (pp. 103–118). New York: Winston-Wiley.

House, R. J. (1971). A path-goal theory of leader effectiveness. *Administrative Science Quarterly, 16*, 321–338.

Jago, A. G. (1982). Perspectives in theory and research. *Management Science, 28*, 315–336.

Jones, J. M., Meredith, S., Wadas, L., Watt, S., & Weisz, E. (1991). The contribution and role of the social worker. In National Advisory Council on Aging (Ed.), *Geriatric assessment and treatment: Members of the team* (pp. 35–52). No. H71–2/1–1991E. Ottawa, ON: Minister of Supply and Services Canada.

Kaluzny, A. (1985). Design and management of disciplinary and interdisciplinary groups in health services: Review and critique. *Medical Care Review, 42*, 77–112.

Kane, R. A. (1975). *Interprofessional teamwork* (Manpower Monograph No. 8). Syracuse, NY: Syracuse University School of Social Work.

Kappelman, M. M., Bartnick, L. A., Cahn, B., & Rapoport, M. I. (1981). A non-traditional geriatric teaching model: Interprofessional service/education sites. *Journal of Medical Education, 56*, 467–477.

Katz, D., & Kahn, R. L. (1978). *The social psychology of organizations* (2nd ed.). New York: Wiley.

Kaufman, S. R. (1986). *The ageless self: Sources of meaning in late life*. Madison: University of Wisconsin Press.

Kaufman, S. R. (1995). Decision making, responsibility, and advocacy in geriatric medicine: Physician dilemmas with elderly in the community. *The Gerontologist, 35*, 481–488.

Kayser-Jones, J. S. (1986). Distributive justice and the treatment of acute illness in nursing homes. *Social Science in Medicine, 23*, 1279–1286.

Kolb, D. A. (1984). *Experiental learning*. Englewood Cliffs, NJ: Prentice-Hall.

Kramer, R. M. & Tyler, T. R. (1996). *Trust in organizations. Frontiers of theory and research*. Thousand Oaks, CA: Sage.

Lacoursiere, R. B. (1980). *The life cycle of groups: Group development stage theory*. New York: Human Sciences Press.

Leape, L. L. (1994). Error in medicine. *Journal of the American Medical Association, 272*, 1851–1857.

Lewin, K. R., Lippitt, R., & White, R. K. (1939). Patterns of aggressive behavior in experimentally created social climates. *Journal of Social Psychology, 10*, 271–299.

Lombardo, M. M. (1978). *Looking at leadership: Some neglected issues* (Tech. Rep. No. 6). Greensboro, NC: Center for Creative Leadership.

Lowe, J. I., & Herranen, M. (1978). Conflict in teamwork: Understanding roles and relationships. *Social Work in Health Care, 3*, 323–330.

Lowe, J. I., & Herranen, M. (1981). Understanding teamwork: Another look at the concepts. *Social Work in Health Care, 7*(2), 1–11.

Mailick, M. D., & Ashley, A. A. (1981). Politics of interprofessional collaboration: Challenge to advocacy. *Social Casework, 62*, 131–137.

McCall, M. W., Jr., & Lombardo, M. M. (Eds.). (1982). *Leadership: Where else can we go?* Durham, NC: Duke University Press.

McClelland, M., & Sands, R. G. (1993). The missing voice in interdisciplinary communication. *Qualitative Health Research, 3*, 74–90.

Mishler, E. G. (1984). *The discourse of medicine: Dialectics of medical interviews*. Norwood, NJ: Ablex.

Mizrahi, T. (1984). Managing medical mistakes: Ideology, insularity and accountability among internists-in-training. *Social Science and Medicine, 19*, 135–146.

Mizrahi, T. (1986). *Getting rid of patients: Contradictions in the socialization of physicians*. New Brunswick, NJ: Rutgers University Press.

Mizrahi, T., & Abramson, J. (1985). Sources of strain between physicians and social workers: Implications for social workers in health care settings. *Social Work in Health Care, 10*(3), 33–51.

Morgan, G. (1989). *Creative organization theory*. Newbury Park, CA: Sage.

Morgan, G. (1997). *Images of organization* (2nd ed.). Thousand Oaks, CA: Sage.

Morrissey, S., Moore, S., Cox, G., Queiro-Tajalli, I., & Martz, B. L. (1989). Building interdisciplinary teams in gerontological education. *Educational Gerontology, 15*, 385–394.

Netting, F. E., & Williams, F. G. (1996). Case manager–physician collaboration: Implications for professional identity, roles, and relationships. *Health and Social Work, 21*, 216–224.

Netting, F. E., & Williams, F. G. (1997, March 8). *Preparing the next generation of geriatric social workers to collaborate with primary care physicians*. Paper presented at the annual meeting of the Council on Social Work Education, Chicago, IL.

Orsburn, J. D., Moran, L., Musselwhite, E., & Zenger, J. H. (1990). *Self-directed work teams: The new American challenge*. Homewood, IL: Business One Irwin.

Oshry, B. (1996). *Seeing systems*. San Francisco: Berrett-Koehler.

Parse, R. R. (1987). *Nursing science: Major paradigms, theories, and critiques*. Philadelphia: W. B. Saunders.

Parse, R. R. (1992). Human becoming: Parse's theory of nursing. *Nursing Science Quarterly, 5*, 35–42.

Parsons, T. (1960). *Structure and process in modern societies*. New York: The Free Press.

Perry, W. G. (1970). *Forms of intellectual and ethical development in the college years: A scheme*. New York: Holt, Rinehart & Winston, Inc.

Petrie, H. G. (1976). Do you see what I see? The epistemology of interdisciplinary inquiry. *Journal of Aesthetic Education, 10*, 29–43.

Pfeffer, J. (1981). *Power in organizations*. Marshfield, MA: Pitman.

Potter, R. B. (1969). *War and moral discourse*. Richmond, VA: John Knox Press.

Qualls, S. H., & Czirr, R. (1988). Geriatric health teams: Classifying models of professional and team functioning. *The Gerontologist, 28*, 372–376.

Quinn, R. E., & Walsh, J. P. (1994). Understanding organizational tragedies: The case of the Hubble space telescope. *Academy of Management Executive, 8*, 62–67.

Ray, D., & Bronstein, H. (1995). *Teaming up: Making the transition to a self-directed team-based organization*. New York: McGraw-Hill.

Reiser, S. J. (1993). The era of the patient: Using the experience of illness in shaping the missions of health care. *Journal of the American Medical Association, 269*, 1012–1017.

Risse, G. B. (1982). Once on top, now on tap: American physicians view their relationships with patients, 1920–1970. In G. J. Agich (Ed.), *Responsibility in health care* (pp. 23–49). Dordrecht, Holland: D. Reidel.

Rittel, H., & Webber, M. (1973). Dilemmas in a general theory of planning, *Policy Sciences*, 4, 155–169.

Romig, D. A. (1996). *Breakthrough teamwork*. Chicago, IL: Irwin.

Roter, D. L., & Hall, J. A. (1992). *Doctors talking with patients/patients talking with doctors*. Westport, CT: Auburn House.

Salancik, G. J., & Pfeffer, J. (1977). Who gets power—and how they hold on to it: A strategic contingency model of power. *Organizational Dynamics, 5*, 3–21.

Sampson, E. E., & Marthas, M. (1990). *Group process for the health professions* (3rd ed.). Albany, NY: Delmar.

Sands, R. G. (1989). The social worker joins the team: A look at the socialization process. *Social Work in Health Care, 14*(2), 1–14.

Schatzman, L., & Strauss, A. (1973). *Field research: Strategies for a natural sociology*. Englewood Cliffs, NJ: Prentice Hall.

Schmitt, M. H., Farrell, M. P., & Heinemann, G. D. (1988). Conceptual and methodological problems in studying the effects of interdisciplinary geriatric teams. *The Gerontologist, 28*, 53–764.

Schön, D. A. (1984). Leadership as reflection in action. In T. J. Sergiovanni & J. E. Corbally (Eds.), *Leadership and organizational culture: New perspectives on administrative theory and practice* (pp. 36–63). Chicago: University of Illinois Press.

Schön, D. A. (1987). *Educating the reflective practitioner*. San Francisco, CA: Jossey-Bass.

Seed, A. (1994). Patients to people. *Journal of Advanced Nursing, 19*, 738–748.

Self, D. J., Schrader, D. E., Baldwin, D. C., & Wolinsky, F. D. (1991). A pilot study of the relationship of medical education and moral development. *Academic Medicine, 66*, 629.

Siegler, E. L., Hyer, K., Fulmer, T., & Mezey, M. (1998). *Geriatric interdisciplinary team training*. New York: Springer.

Siegler, E. L., & Whitney, F. W. (1994). *Nurse–physician collaboration: Care of adults and the elderly*. New York: Springer.

Silver, G. (1958). Beyond general practice: The health team. *Yale Journal of Biology and Medicine, 31*, 29–38.

Smith, K. K., & Berg, D. N. (1987). *Paradoxes of group life*. San Francisco: Jossey-Bass.

Smith, P. B., & Peterson, M. F. (1988). *Leadership, organizations, and culture*. London: Sage.

Starr, P. (1982). *The social transformation of American medicine*. New York: Basic Books.

Stein, L. I. (1967). The doctor–nurse game. *Archives of General Psychiatry, 16*, 699–703.

Stein, L. I., Watts, D. T., & Howell, T. (1990). The doctor-nurse game revisited. *The New England Journal of Medicine, 322*, 546–549.

Stetler, C. B., & Charns, M. P. (Eds.) (1995). *Collaboration in health care*. Chicago, IL: American Hospital Publishing.

Stogdill, R. M. (1948). Personal factors associated with leadership: A survey of the literature. *Journal of Psychology, 25*, 35–71.

Stogdill, R. M., & Coons, A. E. (Eds.). (1957). *Leader behavior: Its description and measurement*. Columbus: Bureau of Business Research, The Ohio State University.

Terman, L. M. (1904). A preliminary study of the psychology and pedagogy of leadership. *Journal of Genetic Psychology, 11*, 413–451.

Thomas, K. W. (1977). Toward multi-dimensional values in teaching: The example of conflict behaviors. *Academy of Management Review, 12*, 484–490.

Toner, J. A., Miller, P., & Gurland, B. J. (1994). Conceptual, theoretical, and practical approaches to the development of interdisciplinary teams: A transactional model. *Educational Gerontology, 20*, 53–69.

Tower, K. D. (1994). Consumer-centered social work practice: Restoring client self-determination. *Social Work, 39*, 191–196.

Tsukuda, R. A. (1990). Interdisciplinary collaboration: Teamwork in geriatrics. In C. K. Cassel, D. E. Riesenberg, L. B. Sorenson, & J. R. Walsh (Eds.), *Geriatric medicine* (2nd. ed., pp. 668–675). New York: Springer-Verlag.

Vroom, V. H., & Jago, A. G. (1988). *The new leadership: Managing participation in organizations*. Englewood Cliffs, NJ: Prentice-Hall.

Walker, R. M., Miles, S. H., Stocking, C. B., & Siegler, M. (1991). Physicians' and nurses' perceptions of ethics problems on general medical services. *Journal of General Internal Medicine, 6*, 424–429.

Watts, D. T., McCaulley, B. L., & Priefer, B. A. (1990). Physician-nurse conflict: Lessons from a clinical experience. *Journal of the American Geriatrics Society, 38*, 1151–1152.

Williams, R. A., & Williams, C. C. (1982). Hospital social workers and nurses: Interprofessional perceptions and experiences. *Journal of Nursing Education, 21*(5), 16–21.

Wise, H., Beckhard, R., Rubin, I., & Kyte, A. (1974). *Making health teams work.* Cambridge, MA: Ballinger.

Witman, A. B., Park, D. M., & Hardin, S. B. (1996). How do patients want physicians to handle mistakes. *Archives of Internal Medicine, 156,* 2565–2569.

Wolf, S. M. (1988). Conflict between doctor and patient. *Law, Medicine, and Health Care, 16,* 197–203.

Yukl, G. A. (1981). *Leadership in organizations.* Englewood Cliffs, NJ: Prentice-Hall.

Zeiss, A. M., & Steffen, A. M. (1996). Interdisciplinary health care teams: The basic unit of geriatric care. In L. L. Carstensen, B. A. Edelstein, & L. Dornbrand (Eds.), *The practical handbook of clinical gerontology* (pp. 423–450). Thousand Oaks, CA: Sage.

Index

About the Authors

THERESA J. K. DRINKA worked for 20 years with interdisciplinary health care teams as a clinician, trainer, administrator, and researcher at the University of Wisconsin and the Department of Veterans Affairs. In 1996 she founded River's Edge Consulting and codeveloped Team Signatures, a unique technology that allows trainers to evaluate a team's changing dynamics.

PHILLIP G. CLARK is Professor of Gerontology and the Director of both the Program in Gerontology and the Rhode Island Geriatric Education Center at The University of Rhode Island. He has extensive experience in teaching interdisciplinary health care team courses, developing interdisciplinary health care research and demonstration projects, and consulting on interdisciplinary educational development and evaluation projects in the U.S. and Canada.